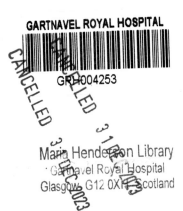
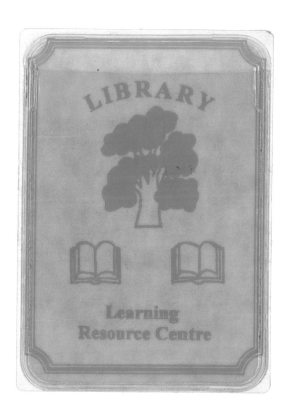

Treating Trichotillomania

SERIES IN ANXIETY AND RELATED DISORDERS

Series Editor: **Martin M. Antony,** *Professor, Department of Psychology,
Ryerson University, Toronto, Ontario, Canada*

A Continuation Order Plan is available for this series. A continuation order will bring delivery of each
new volume immediately upon publication. Volumes are billed only upon actual shipment. For further
information please contact the publisher.

Treating Trichotillomania

Cognitive-Behavioral Therapy for Hairpulling and Related Problems

Martin E. Franklin

University of Pennsylvania School of Medicine
Philadelphia, Pennsylvania, USA

David F. Tolin

Institute of Living/Hartford Hospital
Hartford, Connecticut, USA

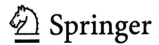 Springer

Martin E. Franklin
Center for the Treatment and Study
   of Anxiety
University of Pennsylvania School
   of Medicine
3535 Market Street
Philadelphia, PA 19104
USA

David F. Tolin
The Institute of Living
The Institute of Living/Hartford
   Hospital
200 Retreat Ave.
Hartford, CT 06106
USA

ISBN-13: 978-0-387-70882-9   e-ISBN-13: 978-0-387-70883-6

Library of Congress Control Number: 2007926594

Printed on acid-free paper.

9 8 7 6 5 4 3 2 1

springer.com

PREFACE

The first and perhaps most important step in writing a treatment manual for use in clinical practice is to clearly explicate the logic of how the treatment, and hence the book, should be organized. Accordingly, our goal in this section is to lay out the structure of cognitive-behavioral therapy (CBT) for trichotillomania (TTM) and other body-focused impulse control disorders, clearly explaining critical decisions such as the chosen sequence of techniques or whether a given technique is considered a core component or a module to be used in some but not all cases. The structure of this particular book is influenced by the work of experts who have gone before us in pioneering CBT for TTM, and is also informed by over a decade of our own clinical work and research on TTM across the developmental spectrum. We are indebted to those who developed this approach to treatment and also to those who built the extant literature on the psychopathology of TTM and related disorders. These clinicians and researchers did so in order to help alleviate the suffering of those afflicted with these conditions, and we endeavor to follow in their footsteps in continuing this important work.

One of the first decisions we needed to make about the book's emphasis was whether to create a treatment guide that focused primarily on the treatment of adult TTM with a separate chapter on developmental adjustments needed to conduct CBT with children and adolescents. We chose not to do this for several reasons: 1) much of our work with TTM in the last decade has been with youth, and we felt that our experiences with this population warranted more discussion than was feasible in a single chapter; 2) although there is a clear need to adapt treatment to the developmental level of the patient, the underlying core principles cut across the developmental spectrum and hence were more efficiently considered together; and 3) TTM is typically a pediatric onset disorder, and thus its treatment should be given equal weight compared to the treatment of adults. We encourage therapists with an interest in CBT for TTM but have worked primarily with adults to consider seeking additional training, supervision, and clinical experience in treating youth: there is a serious problem with treatment access for TTM in general, but this problem is particularly pronounced for families seeking help for their children.

The book is organized into four subsections: 1) Overview and Assessment; 2) Treatment: Core Elements; 3) Treatment: Adjunctive Modules; and 4) Resources for Clinicians, Patients, and Families. We encourage readers to delve into the descriptive details of TTM presented in the first section, before attempting to use the core treatment techniques, since TTM is a heterogeneous disorder in which one clinical presentation does not necessarily inform the clinician about the particulars of the next case. It is also clear that initial assessments with TTM patients are much more likely to go smoothly if the therapist demonstrates comprehensive knowledge of the ins and outs of TTM, such as the common behavioral, environmental, and affective antecedents to pulling, likely pulling sites, and the presence of post-pulling behaviors such as rolling the pulled hair between the thumb and index finger, chewing the root, and visually inspecting the hair, to name but a few. It is often reassuring to patients and families when the therapist demonstrates this kind of ready familiarity with TTM – many of our own patients and their families have reported that they themselves had to educate prior medical and mental health professionals with whom they had contact about the nature of TTM, and thus it is comforting to meet a therapist with extensive knowledge about TTM. Full awareness about the details of TTM is also critically important in devising a treatment plan that is properly tailored. Here again, detailed knowledge about the nature of TTM, which is emphasized in the first section of the book, will likely come in handy in formulating questions to elicit the necessary information about the specifics of a given patient's pulling behavior. We recommend against the use of this (or any other) treatment manual as a "cookbook," in which specific interventions are selected based solely on the patient's diagnosis; rather, think of this manual as an aid to designing your own treatments, tailored to meet the needs of each individual patient.

The book's second section describes what we consider to be the core elements of CBT for TTM, and these chapters are presented in the order in which we typically present the techniques in clinical practice and in our recently completed CBT development project for pediatric TTM which was funded by the National Institute of Mental Health (NIMH). The presentation of maintenance techniques following the implementation of the treatment procedures requires no further explanation, and it is similarly clear that awareness training is needed up front to identify the high-risk situations and affective states that prompt pulling; without this information, implementation of stimulus control and competing response techniques would likely prove unhelpful. The ordering of stimulus control and habit reversal requires more consideration, however. We typically find that more information is needed about the function of pulling in order to properly select competing responses tailored to the specific needs of a given patient, whereas stimulus control methods primarily require knowledge of high-risk situations, information that is more readily available from the initial intake and from early self-monitoring efforts, and thus we recommend that stimulus control methods be taught and implemented before beginning competing response training.

In the third section of the book we include several modules that can be used on an "as needed" basis, and within those chapters we endeavor to describe in great detail what kinds of clinical situations may warrant their inclusion. Notably, many prior CBT books (including our own) had included relaxation and cognitive restructuring techniques as part of the core treatment to be implemented with every patient, but data from our CBT development project as well as observations of other experts suggested that they may not be necessary for everyone. We conducted pilot CBT study for pediatric TTM as part of the NIMH project in which we did just that, but we also collected data about utilization of techniques and patient satisfaction with specific techniques. With our colleague Gretchen Diefenbach, we conducted similar data with adults receiving CBT. These data and our clinical impressions from treating numerous children, adolescents, and adults suggested that patients did not appear to like or use relaxation and cognitive restructuring very much, whereas the other techniques of awareness training, stimulus control, and competing response training were received more favorably and used more often (Brady, Diefenbach, Tolin, Hannan & Crocetto, 2005; Tolin, Franklin, & Diefenbach, 2002). We removed these techniques from the core protocol for the subsequent randomized controlled trial that was conducted as part of the NIMH pediatric project, and results with the more streamlined protocol were very promising (Franklin, Roth Ledley, Cardona, Anderson, & Hajcak, 2005). Thus, we encourage therapists to take this same approach, and we make specific recommendations in the chapter about when to consider adding these particular modules. We also chose to include modules on managing psychiatric comorbidity, family problems, and motivational enhancement, each of which can pose significant challenges to successful implementation of the core treatment. We also included a module on group-based approaches, which may prove especially helpful in situations where professional resources are limited.

The book's final section includes information about resources available to therapists, patients, and families alike, and hopefully continuing progress in the field will assure that our collection of such materials will be rendered incomplete in due time. One particularly helpful resource is the Trichotillomania Learning Center, an organization that has been in the vanguard when it comes to informing the lay and professional communities about TTM and its treatment. With her seemingly endless supply of enthusiasm and caring, TLC's Executive Director, Christina Pearson, has assured the continuing relevance of TLC in the struggle to improve the lives of those who have TTM themselves or have a loved one with the disorder. Christina has been a major inspiration to this project and, indeed, for much of our work in TTM.

Finally, we wish to emphasize that truly informed treatment development requires input from the clinical researchers who develop the protocols, patients, and family members, as well as the front-line clinicians who implement the treatments in clinical contexts where most families can access care. We therefore encourage mental health professionals who purchase this guide and begin to use it in clinical practice to contact us with their comments, critiques, and suggestions (marty@mail.med.upenn.edu and dtolin@harthosp.org). The book, as well as our conceptual understanding of TTM and its treatment more broadly, are very much works in progress, and accordingly we seek as much help with understanding the strengths and limitations of this book as we can get. Both of the authors are notable for the thickness of their skin, and are therefore likely to carefully consider feedback regardless of its valence.

ACKNOWLEDGEMENTS

We began treating individuals with trichotilllomania (TTM) at the Medical College of Pennsylvania's Center for the Treatment and Study of Anxiety (CTSA), which later moved to the University of Pennsylvania School of Medicine. We both learned a tremendous amount from our CTSA colleagues, and want to acknowledge them all for their willingness to help us better understand TTM and its impact—in particular, the CTSA's Director, Edna Foa. Many colleagues were exceptionally helpful in our TTM research projects, and although there is not enough space to acknowledge them all by name, we do want to thank Donald Bux, Shawn Cahill, Kelly Chrestman, Gretchen Diefenbach, Michael Kozak, Deborah Roth Ledley, Suzanne Meunier, Kim Treadwell, Elna Yadin, and Lori Zoellner, who greatly informed and shaped our thinking about TTM and related disorders. We also wish to acknowledge the efforts of Sharon Panulla and Marty Antony, our editor and the series editor, respectively. They encouraged us, supported us, and kept us on task; their wise counsel and boundless patience allowed us to create a book that we hope bridges the gap between science and clinical practice.

We would also like to acknowledge the tremendous support given to us by the Trichotillomania Learning Center (TLC) and its Director, Christina Pearson. Our involvement with TLC and with Christina has enriched us both professionally and personally. Through our affiliation with TLC we have also had the great fortune of developing collaborative relationships with many of the leaders in the field of TTM clinical and research, including Doug Woods, Nancy Keuthen, Charlie Mansueto, Suzanne Mouton-Odum, Fred Penzel, John Piacentini, and others. We have learned much of what we now know about TTM and its treatment from the experts we've met through TLC, and their influence can be seen throughout this volume. And, of course, we thank the many adults, adolescents and children with TTM and related disorders who have participated in our research projects, come to our clinics, or talked to us at meetings and conferences. They have been our very best teachers, and this book is dedicated to them.

MEF and DFT

Ten years ago I had barely heard of trichotillomania (TTM). As a new clinician and researcher, my interests at that time lay in the area of obsessive-compulsive disorder (OCD) and other anxiety-related conditions. I started working with a new colleague named Marty Franklin, who not only helped shape my thinking about OCD, but also shared with me his interest in TTM. Needless to say, he got my attention, and I'm glad he did. It's been a pleasure and privilege to learn about, study, and treat adults and adolescents struggling with this disorder. My graduate school mentors, Jeff Lohr and Ron Kleinknecht, helped set me on the path that eventually led to this project. I am grateful to the Institute of Living for supporting my work, and particularly to my colleagues at the Anxiety Disorders Center for all of their hard work and enthusiasm. And to Fiona, James, and Catherine—thanks for your love and patience.

DFT

I have been incredibly fortunate in that I have received great mentorship throughout my academic pursuits, including Fr. Charles Lemkuhl, S.J., Douglas Klieger, Trish Morokoff, and Jim Curran during my undergraduate and graduate school years, and Edna Foa, Michael Kozak, and John March since then. I am also eternally grateful for the enthusiastic support of my sisters Margaret, Marie, and Maud, who vigorously encourage me to take risks such as book writing, and to our parents Domnick and Kay Franklin for the many sacrifices they have made on our behalf. Finally I wish to thank my wife Marlene Gawarkiewicz, who had faith in me long before I did and has provided boundless support, friendship, and love for the last two decades – I am truly the luckiest man on the face of the earth. I also want to thank our three children, Gwendolyn (10), Delia (7), and Teddy (2), who at times have had to tolerate my long hours at the expense of a game of catch, reading a fun book, or watching a movie as a family. In fact, Delia's cogent comment on the penultimate draft of this manuscript helped hasten its completion: "Daddy, haven't you written enough words *yet*?" Hopefully by now we have, and hopefully these words will prove useful to you in your own work with individuals with TTM.

MEF

CONTENTS

Part 2: TREATMENT: CORE ELEMENTS

Part 3: TREATMENT: ADJUNCTIVE MODULES
Introduction to Part 3: Modules

PART 1

OVERVIEW AND ASSESSMENT

CHAPTER 1

TRICHOTILLO-WHAT?

Definition, Epidemiology, & Impairment

DEFINITION OF TTM

Trichotillomania (TTM) is a chronic impulse control disorder characterized by pulling out of one's own hair, resulting in noticeable hair loss. The syndrome has been described in the psychiatric annals as far back as the 19th century, yet research on its epidemiology, psychopathology, and treatment remains scarce. TTM has received increased attention in the last decade, culminating with the publication of the first textbook devoted entirely to the disorder (Stein, Christenson, & Hollander, 1999).

According to the DSM IV-TR (American Psychiatric Association, 2000), a diagnosis of TTM requires:

A) Recurrent pulling out of one's hair resulting in noticeable hair loss.
B) An increasing sense of tension immediately before pulling out the hair or when attempting to resist the behavior.
C) Pleasure, gratification or relief when pulling out the hair.
D) The disturbance is not better accounted for by another mental disorder and not due to a general medical condition (e.g., a dermatological condition).
E) The disturbance causes clinically significant distress or impairment in social, occupational, or other important areas of functioning.

A key feature of the DSM-IV-TR diagnosis is that patients experience increasing tension prior to pulling, which is subsequently relieved by pulling. Criteria B and C are somewhat controversial, given that a significant minority of adults who pull their hair do not report experiencing these criteria. In a sample of 60 adult patients, 5% failed to endorse a feeling of tension prior to pulling, and 12% did not report gratification or tension release subsequent to pulling (Christenson, MacKenzie, & Mitchell, 1991); similarly, Schlosser, Black, Blum, and Goldstein (1994) indicated that 23% of their clinical sample failed to meet the diagnostic criteria of tension and gratification. Moreover, the applicability of DSM IV Criteria B and C may be even more tenuous in youth. For example, only half of a small sample of children and adolescents endorsed both rising tension and relief associated with hair pulling (Hanna, 1997), whereas endorsement of these symptoms appears more common in older children and adolescents (King, Scahill et al., 1995). This pattern might be due to developmentally appropriate differences between young children and adults with respect to their ability to describe their state of mind prior to engaging in pulling behavior and the psychological effects of pulling. In both adult and pediatric samples, some patients describe a pattern of "focused" pulling, in which they are aware of the behavior and its impact on their emotional state, whereas others engage in "unfocused" pulling, in which they are not aware (or only dimly aware) of how they are feeling or even the fact that they are pulling. This distinction will be discussed in greater detail later. On the whole, findings on the DSM IV criteria for TTM suggest that the current diagnostic classification scheme may be overly restrictive. Accordingly, many outcome researchers who are studying TTM do not require that participants endorse Criteria B and/or C. In our own work we have been somewhat flexible regarding the full diagnostic criteria: if a patient is pulling enough to result in noticeable alopecia, the pulling is not better accounted for by another condition, and the pulling is causing significant distress or impairment, we typically will still consider the patient further for entry into treatment programs and clinical research studies. Little research has been done to examine differences between those who meet full diagnostic criteria and those who do not, and thus many unanswered questions remain about whether or not these should be considered the same syndrome.

DESCRIPTIVE FEATURES OF TTM

One of the first things that struck us as we began to work clinically with TTM patients was the heterogeneity of the disorder. Although the common features identified in the DSM-IV-TR definition of TTM give the clinician some expectation of what TTM is, there appears to be so much variety in terms of descriptive psychopathology that it raises the question as to whether TTM could possibly have a single etiological factor. Our view is that TTM is multi-determined, serving different functions for different people; and that discovery of the function of TTM for each individual patient is critical to the development of a successful CBT strategy. Below, we describe some of the more common variants of pulling that are likely to be encountered with TTM. We also find that asking about TTM at this level of detail early on in the assessment sessions can increase the patient and/or family's confidence that the therapist is truly informed about the nature of the condition, which then decreases shame about sharing details about pulling that many of these patients have not previously shared with others. We discuss this aspect of the initial clinical interviews in detail in Chapters 3 and 4 of this volume.

PULLING SITES

Scalp hair is the most common pulling site in adults (Christenson, MacKenzie et al., 1991; Lerner, Franklin, Meadows, Hembree, & Foa, 1998), with eyelashes and eyebrows being the next most frequently reported pulling site. However, all body hair is potentially vulnerable, as some TTM patients pull from pubic areas, trunk, arms, legs, beard, chest, etc. Notably, over one third of a recent clinical sample reported pulling from more than one site (Lerner et al., 1998), so it is important to inquire about other sites even when a patient's alopecia or methods of covering bald patches makes it clear that the patient is pulling from the scalp and/or eyelashes and eyebrows.

Less information is available on how TTM presents in children and adolescents, but the data that are available are convergent with information about clinical features of adult hair-pulling: the scalp appears to be the most common pulling site in children and adolescents, followed by eyelashes and eyebrows (Reeve, 1999). We (Tolin, Franklin, Diefenbach, Anderson, & Meunier, 2006) found that 11 of 47 (23%) children and adolescents pulled from two or more sites, 23 (49%) pulled scalp hair exclusively, and 13 (28%) pulled eyelashes exclusively. Nearly a third of children reported that the site of pulling had changed over time. The absence of body hair on younger children precludes pulling from certain sites, but clinical work with adolescents appears consistent with the adult data in that pulling from sites other than the face and scalp is also common.

There is little information about whether the preferred pulling site is predictive of treatment outcome, psychiatric comorbidity, or of other descriptive features of TTM such as whether the pulling behavior is fully conscious, but certainly the relative number of hairs on the scalp as opposed to the eyelashes and eyebrows does raise clinically relevant issues. Because there are relatively fewer eyelashes and eyebrows compared to scalp hair, a large percentage of the pulling site can be denuded quickly when eyebrows and eyelashes are involved, and the resultant damage can be more difficult to conceal. This issue comes up in treatment a fair amount and will be discussed in subsequent chapters; our concern is that the large amount of hair removal in a short period of time can be demoralizing, and thus has implications for motivation to work on the hair pulling in any sort of concerted way.

HAIR REMOVAL METHODS

Hairs are usually pulled one at a time using the thumb and index or middle finger on the dominant hand, although we have also encountered patients who describe a progression from pulling one at a time close to the root to grabbing several hairs at the ends and pulling them out simultaneously. Some patients use implements such as tweezers to remove hair, while others rub the hair until it is broken from the root. These examples are neither exhaustive nor mutually exclusive, however, which underscores the importance of asking specifically about the method of hair extraction and querying the patient as to whether the preferred method is the only one used or whether there are times when other means are attempted.

HAIR SELECTION

A majority of patients describe searching for hairs with certain textural qualities (Christenson, MacKenzie et al., 1991); relatively fewer pull in response to visual cues such as hair of differing length than the majority of hair, gray hair, etc. For patients with strong visual cues or who pull from sites unlikely to be exposed in public (e.g., pubic hair), time spent isolated in bathrooms is particularly risky, especially for patients with pre-pulling visual inspection rituals who have access to brightly lit bathrooms. Patients often describe touching or stroking their hair prior to engaging in pulling. There might be an interaction between pulling site and hair selection in that those who pull eyelashes or eyebrows might be more likely to have visual cues that prompt pulling, although this is speculative. Nevertheless, it is important to consider the way that a patient makes the hair selection as you develop a comprehensive treatment plan, as the implementation of stimulus control methods will be determined in part by this feature.

POST-PULLING BEHAVIORS

Once a hair is pulled, patients vary with respect to additional behaviors such as manipulating the hair in their hands, placing it in their mouths, inspecting the hair and its root, or eating the hair. Some patients simply discard the pulled hair and quickly continue pulling additional hairs. Most patients can identify high risk situations for pulling such as isolated time in the bathroom, talking on the phone, watching television, driving, reading, or immediately prior to falling asleep. Triggers may vary depending on whether the patient is primarily a focused or unfocused puller. Certain affective states, such as boredom, frustration, anxiety, and sadness, can also serve as cues for pulling (see Chapter 2). Clinically, we have found it helpful at intake to describe to patients some of the common presentations of TTM. Provision of such information helps patients overcome the embarrassment and shame they feel in discussing the details of their pulling behavior.

FOCUSED VERSUS UNFOCUSED PULLING

Approximately 75% of adult TTM patients report that most of their hair-pulling behavior takes place "automatically" or outside of awareness (i.e., unfocused pulling), whereas the remaining 25% describe themselves as primarily focused on hair-pulling when they pull (i.e., focused pulling) (Christenson & MacKenzie, 1994). Some researchers have postulated that TTM patients who engage primarily in focused hair-pulling are more "OCD-like" and also may be more responsive to pharmacological interventions found effective for OCD (e.g., Christenson & O'Sullivan, 1996). However, the distinction between focused and unfocused pullers is complicated by the fact that at least some patients engage in both types of pulling behavior. Clinically, we have observed that patients who engage in both types of pulling often progress from unfocused pulling of a few hairs which strengthens the urge to pull, then is followed by focused pulling. Assessment of both types of pulling behavior is imperative prior to beginning a CBT program because clinical intervention strategies will differ depending on whether focused or unfocused pulling is primary.

As children get older, there appears to be a fairly predictable association between hair-pulling and relatively sedentary activities (Reeve, 1999); hair-pulling during such activities is also characteristic of unfocused pulling in adults. Thus, awareness training (see Chapter 7) is likely to be a critical intervention in treatment for children and adolescents who engage primarily in unfocused pulling, less so with focused pullers. CBT for TTM must be sufficiently flexible to address the various forms of TTM, including focused and unfocused pulling.

EPIDEMIOLOGY OF TTM

Large-scale, methodologically adequate epidemiological surveys of TTM have not been attempted in either adult or pediatric samples, so the true prevalence of these problems remains undocumented. However, the smaller-scale survey data that are available suggest that TTM is much more prevalent than previously reported (e.g., Adam & Kashani, 1990). In a community-based prevalence study of 218 adults, 4% of those surveyed reported current or past hair pulling in a manner consistent with TTM, although not necessarily meeting diagnostic criteria (Graber & Arndt, 1993). Christenson, Pyle, and Mitchell (1991) reported a 0.6% lifetime prevalence rate for DSM-III-R (American Psychiatric Association, 1987) TTM (which did not include the tension criterion) in a college sample. When hair pulling not meeting full diagnostic criteria was estimated in this sample, prevalence rates increased to 1.5% for males and 3.4% for females. Consistent with these estimates, Rothbaum, Shaw, Morris, and Ninan (1993) found that 11% of a college sample reported some hair pulling and 2% reported pulling with visible hair loss; and King, Zohar et al. (1995) estimated a lifetime hair pulling prevalence rate of 1% among 17-year-olds. However, the generalization of these data to more representative epidemiological research is unclear, and there remains a need for epidemiological research on TTM.

IMPACT OF TTM

TTM is often associated with significant emotional, social, and medical problems. In addition to the time spent on hair pulling itself, many sufferers spend considerable time concealing large resultant bald areas (Swedo & Leonard, 1992), and experience guilt, shame, and low self-esteem (Diefenbach, Tolin, Hannan, Crocetto, & Worhunsky, 2005; Stanley & Mouton, 1996). The disorder can also lead to avoidance of activities in which hair loss might be exposed (e.g., swimming), avoidance of activities that may lead to direct physical contact with others (e.g., intimate relationships, sports) and, in more extreme cases, complete social isolation (Winchel, Jones, Molcho et al., 1992). Because TTM usually strikes during sensitive developmental years, it can be especially disabling (Rothbaum & Ninan, 1994). Children and adolescents who develop TTM often become extremely self-conscious of the effects of hair pulling on their appearance, and go to great lengths to avoid many typical childhood activities in order to maintain secrecy about the disorder. Sometimes this avoidant strategy results in their receiving fewer invitations to participate in future activities, which compounds their sense of isolation. Moreover, when peers discover evidence of their pulling inadvertently, these youngsters often experience a great sense of shame and embarrassment that clearly impacts social relationships. Adolescents are particularly vulnerable to negative feedback from their peer group, and discovery of a secret such as TTM can be especially difficult on them.

PSYCHIATRIC COMORBIDITY

In addition to the problems resulting directly from the hair pulling itself, psychiatric comorbidity appears to be common in adults seeking treatment for TTM. Christenson, MacKenzie et al. (1991) found that 82% of their TTM sample met criteria for a past or current comorbid Axis I disorder. For those patients with comorbid diagnoses, there was a lifetime prevalence rate of 65% for mood disorders, 57% for anxiety disorders, 22% for substance use disorders, and 20% for eating disorders. A second study of the same patients indicated that 42% met DSM-III-R criteria for a personality disorder (Christenson, Chernoff-Clementz, & Clementz, 1992). In a larger evaluation of 186 adults seeking treatment for chronic hair-pulling (Christenson, 1995), high rates of comorbidity were again evident, with major depression (57%), generalized anxiety disorder (27%), eating disorders (20%), and alcohol (19%) and other substance abuse (16%) being the most common comorbid conditions.

Less is known about comorbidity in pediatric samples, and what has been found thus far in the few studies that have been conducted is inconsistent. In a mixed sample of children, adolescents, and adults with TTM, Swedo and Leonard (1992) found high rates of comorbidity for unipolar depression (39%), generalized anxiety disorder (32%), OCD (16%), and substance abuse (15%). In pediatric clinical samples, Reeve, Bernstein and Christenson (1992) and King, Scahill et al. (1995) found that 7 of 10 (70%) and 9 of 15 (60%) children with TTM had at least one comorbid Axis I disorder, respectively. In the Reeve et al. (1992) study, overanxious disorder was the most commonly diagnosed comorbid condition; in the King et al. (1995) study, disruptive behavior disorders were more common. Conversely, we (Tolin et al., 2006) found that only 18 of 48 (38%) of our child and adolescent sample met criteria for a comorbid disorder. Sampling issues most likely underlie the reduced comorbidity rate, in that our samples were subject to a telephone screen up front that may have excluded some cases likely to evidence severe comorbid psychopathology. Like Reeve et al. (1992), we found that anxiety disorders were the most common comorbid conditions (29%), particularly generalized anxiety disorder (12%). Externalizing disorders (10%), depressive disorders (8%), and tic disorders (2%) were less frequently diagnosed. In contrast with the hypothesized relationship between OCD and TTM (see below), only 6% of our TTM sample met diagnostic criteria for OCD—more than would be expected in the general population, but hardly a large overlap.

QUALITY OF LIFE/FUNCTIONAL IMPAIRMENT

We have described above some of the ways in which TTM can negatively affect emotional and social functioning. Significant rates of avoidance and distress involving public activities, sexual intimacy, and athletic endeavors have been reported in clinical samples (e.g., Diefenbach, Tolin, Hannan et al., 2005; Stemberger, Thomas, Mansueto, & Carter, 2000), and other studies have indicated that many TTM patients spend over one hour per day extracting hair (Koran, Ringold, & Hewlett, 1992; Mansueto, 1990). That said, the systematic study of the effects of TTM on psychosocial functioning using psychometrically sound instruments has only recently begun. Functional limitations were examined in a cohort of adult hair pullers (n = 58) attending the TLC's national conference using survey questions and standardized self-report scales (Keuthen et al., 2002). Seventy-one percent of the sample endorsed TTM-related distress or impairment in social functioning including: decreased contact with friends (40%), decreased dating activity (47%), loss of intimacy (40%), and negative impact on family relationships (50%). In addition, 55% of the sample endorsed TTM-related distress or impairment in occupational functioning including: job avoidance (29%), lateness to work (22%), decreased coworker contact (28%), and decreased career aspirations (34%). Lastly, 69% of the sample endorsed avoidance of specific leisure activities. The Medical Outcomes Study 36-Item Short-Form Health Survey (SF-36; Ware & Sherbourne, 1992) reflected quality of life impairment on all mental health subscales. Severity of hair pulling was negatively correlated with scores on all four subscales and, importantly, depression was found to mediate the relationship between TTM and QOL. Of note, Koran, Thienemann, and Davenport (1996) also reported lowered and comparable quality of life scores for the same SF-36 subscales for an OCD sample in comparison with population norms, further suggesting that the effects of TTM on QOL are far from trivial. In a comparison with nonclinical and clinical control groups, Diefenbach and colleagues (2005) found that both TTM patients and psychiatric controls reported reduced quality of life and social adjustment, as well as increased impairment in occupational, social, and familial functioning. The relationship between TTM and reduced quality of life appeared to be mediated by depression, suggesting that TTM patients' impairment was at least partially the result of comorbid depressed mood. However, even when controlling for depression, the severity of hair pulling and the degree of alopecia predicted poorer functional status and lower quality of life. Specific reported impairments from TTM in that study are shown in Table 1.1. Of note, 100% of patients reported some form of social impairment, 100% reported negative affect, 93% reported grooming-related impairment, 86% reported problems related to physical health, 79% reported reduced productivity, and 68% reported avoidance of recreational activities. Thus, the reductions in quality of life in TTM patients appear profound. Little work of this kind has been done in pediatric hair-pullers, where the presence and impact of teasing related to noticeable hair loss will be especially important to consider.

Table 1.1. Endorsement of Lifetime and Current Interference from Trichotillomania (N=28)

		Lifetime	Past Week
Grooming	Any	26 (92.9%)	24 (85.7%)
	Wear wig, hat, etc.	12 (42.9%)	10 (35.7%)
	Fix hair style a certain way	19 (67.9%)	11 (39.3%)
	Special make-up	11 (39.3%)	9 (32.1%)
	Avoid hairdressers	12 (42.9%)	4 (14.3%)
Physical Health	Any	24 (85.7%)	18 (64.3%)
	Avoid doctors	11 (39.3%)	0
	Eat hair-stomach upset	6 (21.4%)	4 (14.3%)
	Broken skin	6 (21.4%)	3 (10.7%)
	Skin infections	4 (14.3%)	0
	Bleeding	13 (46.4%)	5 (17.9%)
	Scars	5 (17.9%)	3 (10.7%)
	Muscle pain	16 (57.1%)	10 (35.7%)
	Skin irritation	17 (60.7%)	10 (35.7%)
Social Interaction	Any	28 (100%)	27 (96.4%)
	Avoid dating	8 (28.6%)	3 (10.7%)
	Sex life inhibited	6 (21.4%)	4 (14.3%)
	Avoid group social events	8 (28.6%)	1 (3.6%)
	Arguments	7 (25.0%)	0
	Less time with others	9 (32.1%)	5 (17.9%)
	Spend more time alone	9 (32.1%)	6 (21.4%)
	Kept hair pulling a secret	28 (100%)	26 (92.9%)
Recreational Activities	Any	19 (67.9%)	21 (75.0%)
	Avoid swimming	13 (46.4%)	1 (3.6%)
	Avoid other activities	8 (28.6%)	3 (10.7%)
	No activity on windy days	7 (25.0%)	2 (7.1%)
	Less time on things I enjoy	11 (39.3%)	7 (25.0%)
	Avoid sitting in front rows	6 (21.4%)	2 (7.1%)
	Avoid brightly lit rooms	8 (28.6%)	2 (7.1%)
Work Productivity	Any	22 (78.6%)	20 (71.4%)
	Less productive at home	10 (35.7%)	9 (32.1%)
	Less productive at work	7 (25.0%)	6 (21.4%)
	Concentration Problems	17 (60.7%)	15 (53.6%)
	Late for work, appointments, etc.	7 (25.0%)	3 (10.7%)
Negative Affect	Any	28 (100%)	27 (96.4%)
	Feel alone	15 (53.6%)	8 (28.6%)
	Feel "weird" or "strange"	21 (75.0%)	17 (60.7%)
	Feel guilty	18 (64.3%)	14 (50%)
	Feel down on myself	26 (92.9%)	22 (78.6%)
	Feel unattractive	23 (82.1%)	17 (60.7%)
	Had low self-esteem	22 (78.6%)	19 (67.9)
	Worry about hair pulling	24 (85.7%)	20 (71.4%)

From Diefenbach, G. J., Tolin, D. F., Hannan, S., Crocetto, J., & Worhunsky, P. (2005). Trichotillomania: impact on psychosocial functioning and quality of life. *Behaviour Research and Therapy, 43*, 869–884.

ASSOCIATED MEDICAL PROBLEMS

In addition to the social and emotional difficulties described above, as well as substantial psychiatric comorbidity (see Chapter 3), TTM is sometimes associated with significant medical problems such as skin irritation and infections. Indeed, many children and adolescents with TTM are often brought to dermatologists initially, especially when they have not shared the TTM secret with their families. Other medical problems are possible as well. When patients ingest pulled hair (trichophagia), serious gastrointestinal problems stemming from the presence of trichobezoars (packed masses of ingested hairs) also can occur (Swedo & Leonard, 1992; Winchel, Jones, Stanley, Molcho, & Stanley, 1992). Although thought to be uncommon, complications of trichobezoars include gastric or intestinal bleeding, perforation, intestinal obstruction, acute pancreatitis, and obstructive jaundice (Adam & Kashani, 1990; Cardona & Franklin, 2004).

COURSE OF TTM

Adult TTM appears to have its roots in childhood pulling, as the vast majority of adult patients with TTM report onset during late childhood or early adolescence (e.g., Christenson, Pyle et al., 1991). One study of hair pulling courses in a pediatric sample revealed that approximately half of participants reported an intermittent course (symptom-free periods of at least 3 months), with the remaining participants reporting no periods of symptom remission (King et al., 1995). Similarly, we (Tolin et al., 2006) found that 48% of a pediatric sample reported at least one period of complete symptom remission lasting at least two weeks. Meunier, Tolin, Diefenbach, and Brady (2005) asked 35 adult and adolescent (age range 17–57 years) TTM patients to describe their hair-pulling behaviors and associated life events retrospectively over each year of life. Average age of onset was 13 years, with 89% of patients reporting onset during childhood or adolescence. Nearly half (49%) were described as having a chronic course of illness, with no periods of symptom remission and minimal fluctuation in symptom severity. Twenty-nine percent showed a fluctuating course, with multiple fluctuations in severity but no remission. Finally, 23% reported a relapsing and remitting course, with at least one lifetime period of complete symptom remission. Life stressors, particularly major relationship changes, were associated with symptom increase for those with a relapsing and remitting course.

It is not clear whether childhood TTM is a single disorder. Swedo and Leonard (1992) suggest that children with onset prior to age 5, for whom they coined the term "baby trichs," may have a more benign form of the disorder that is likely to resolve without intervention. These young children may engage in pulling behavior as a form of self-soothing, often pulling while trying to fall asleep, sometimes in concert with other self-soothing behaviors such as thumb-sucking or rubbing a favorite stuffed animal or blanket, and possibly under more stressful conditions. In support of the view that there may be a subtype of TTM that differs with respect to presenting symptoms and clinical course, Swedo and Leonard point to the equal ratio of male:female in younger samples in comparison to the predominant female:male ratios observed in clinical samples of adult patients. Clinical work with the families of these very young pullers usually focuses on stress management with the family, with very little focus on the child him/herself or his/her hairpulling (Wright & Holmes, 2003). We will discuss this kind of approach later in the module that addresses family-based interventions.

THE TROUBLE WITH CLASSIFICATION

The inclusion of TTM in DSM-IV-TR among a diverse group of impulse control problems such as intermittent explosive disorder, kleptomania, and pyromania has been criticized as conceptually unfounded (McElroy, Hudson, Pope, Keck, & Aizley, 1992). Some researchers have theorized that TTM is better described as a "nervous habit" with body foci similar to skin picking and nail biting (Christenson & Mansueto, 1999), a class of conditions that will heretofore be referred to as body-focused repetitive behaviors (BFRBs). There seems to be a high prevalence of BFRBs among hair pullers (du Toit, van Kradenburg, Niehaus, & Stein, 2001; Simeon et al., 1997), although the lack of control groups in these studies makes it impossible to determine whether the prevalence of BFRBs is higher in hair pullers than in the general population, where the prevalence of BFRBs is also quite high (Teng, Woods, Twohig, & Marcks, 2002). There is insufficient taxometric data to inform us as to whether TTM and these other BFRBs indeed constitute a theoretically coherent constellation of disorders, and it is therefore unlikely that a new category of BFRBs will emerge as yet. Nevertheless, there are enough similarities clinically that we consider BFRBs from the same theoretical framework that we present later for TTM, and believe there is sufficient preliminary evidence that BFRBs other than TTM respond to the same kinds of CBT interventions that we will discuss in this manual (for a review see Woods & Miltenberger, 2001). Clinically, we tend to use the same basic strategies for treating TTM as we do other BFRBs such as skin-picking, although we note that outcome data, while promising, are sparse (see Deckersbach, Wilhelm, Keuthen, Baer, & Jenike, 2002; Twohig, Hayes, & Masuda, 2006; Twohig & Woods, 2001b).

Related to this is a controversy as to whether TTM and related BFRBs should be considered part of an "OCD spectrum" (Hollander, 1993). Evidence in support of this view includes positive response of TTM patients to clomipramine (Swedo et al., 1989), higher rates of OCD in the family members of individuals with TTM (King, Scahill et al., 1995; Lenane et al., 1992; Tolin et al., 2006), and formal similarities in clinical presentation, as both TTM and OCD involve what patients sometimes describe as compulsive and uncontrollable behaviors (Swedo & Leonard, 1992). Despite these similarities, important differences between the disorders have also been noted. Although some individuals with TTM experience obsessive-type thoughts prior to pulling, the disorder is generally not characterized by the intrusive, repetitive thoughts that are a core symptom of OCD (Stanley & Mouton, 1996; Stanley, Prather, Wagner, Davis, & Swann, 1993; Stanley, Swann, Bowers, Davis, & Taylor, 1992). Furthermore, individuals with TTM typically do not report multiple compulsive behaviors, which is characteristic of OCD (Stanley et al., 1992). Additional evidence suggesting that TTM and OCD are two separate entities is provided by the negative findings for fluoxetine from controlled pharmacological trials (e.g., Christenson, Pyle et al., 1991), and by the findings of Pollard and colleagues (1991) of loss of responsiveness to clomipramine despite continued maintenance on previously effective dosages. Finally, and perhaps most importantly, previous research indicates that individuals with TTM tend to describe their target behavior as pleasurable (Meunier, Tolin, & Franklin, 2005; Stanley et al., 1992), more so than do OCD patients (Stanley et al., 1992), suggesting maintenance of TTM by positive, rather than negative, reinforcement (see Chapter 4). The latter finding is consistent with our clinical observations of most adult and pediatric TTM patients, and therefore our CBT program typically includes efforts to identify and then substitute hair-pulling with an alternative pleasurable activity or behavior.

The question of whether or not to consider TTM to be part of OCD is not merely a nosological abstraction. Because we consider TTM to be functionally distinct from OCD, exposure and response prevention, a highly efficacious treatment for OCD (see Franklin & Foa, 2002; Tolin & Franklin, 2002), is accordingly de-emphasized in our work with TTM: we expect obsessional distress to habituate as a result of prolonged and repeated exposure to anxiety-evoking situations (e.g., contact with a contaminated surface), whereas we have less confidence that urges associated with appetitive behaviors such as TTM will similarly reduce over time with repeated exposure to relevant triggers (e.g., sitting alone in a brightly lit bedroom looking into the mirror). Instead, our CBT for TTM emphasizes awareness training to increase the patient's ability to predict the settings and affective states associated with strong urges to pull, stimulus control methods to block the initiation of pulling because pulling often begins outside of awareness, and competing response training to substitute an alternative activity that provides some of the same positive reinforcement that pulling usually provides. We will discuss each of these core components in detail in the Treatment Section below.

CHAPTER 2

PUTTING IT TOGETHER:

A Biopsychosocial Theory of Trichotillomania and Body-Focused Impulse Control Disorders

In this chapter, we describe a working model of TTM that is also applicable to other BFRBs. As will be described later in this book, researchers and clinicians have developed efficacious psychological and pharmacological treatments for TTM. However, we also recognize that there is much room for growth in this area: although existing treatments can reduce TTM/BFRB symptoms, they often do not eliminate them altogether, and some patients do not maintain their gains over the long term.

We suggest, as have others, that the available treatments are only as good as the empirical model upon which they are based (Foa & Kozak, 1997). Plainly speaking, the more we know about TTM, the more we can "zero in" on its mechanisms with effective interventions. To date, there has not been sufficient study of the psychopathology of TTM or other BFRBs; as a result, our understanding of the factors that cause and/or maintain the disorder is preliminary at best. In this chapter, we present a preliminary biopsychosocial model of TTM, with emphasis on the word "preliminary." We fully expect that over the next decade, as new data are gathered, researchers will add to, subtract from, or replace this model altogether. We look forward to this development and to the enhanced treatment efficacy that is likely to follow. However, for the time being, we find that this model seems to fit our clinical experience, experimental research findings, and the reports of the many people we have met with these disorders. We thank our colleague Gretchen Diefenbach for her assistance in developing this model.

Implied in the very subject of this book is the fact that we consider TTM and BFRB's to be related problems, so much so that they can be condensed into the same broad model and treatment protocol. As we discussed in Chapter 2, there is no clear consensus about whether TTM should be classified as an impulse control disorder or as part of an obsessive-compulsive spectrum, although our belief is that TTM and the BFRBs have more in common with each other (particularly from a behavioral perspective) than they do with OCD. In the meantime, rather than engage in a detailed discussion of whether TTM/BFRBs are part of the obsessive-compulsive spectrum, we have opted here to describe a model of the disorders that will account for biological, psychological, and behavioral findings and hopefully will help the reader to become familiar with the potential mechanisms of the disorders. This model will form the basis of the therapeutic strategies detailed later in this book.

THE MODEL IN BRIEF

Figure 2.1 shows a schematic diagram of our working biopsychosocial model. Many aspects of this model will come as no surprise to readers familiar with biological and cognitive-behavioral underpinnings of behavior; however, for others, some of

Figure 2.1. A Schematic Diagram of a Biopsychosocial Model of Trichotillomania and other Body Focused Impulse Control Disorder.

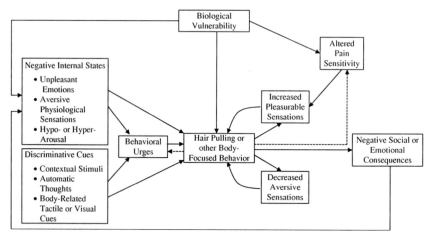

Adapted from Franklin, M. E., Tolin, D.F., & Diefenbach, G.J. (2006). Trichotillomania. In E. Hollander & D.J. Stein (Eds.) *Handbook of impulse control disorders* (pp. 149—173). Washington, DC: American Psychiatric Press.

these components may be novel. The core assumptions of this model and others like it (e.g., Mansueto, Stemberger, Thomas, & Golomb, 1997) are:

- *All behaviors are a product of the pressures and contingencies experienced by the individual.* The implication of this assumption is that all behaviors, no matter how strange, have a logical explanation (even if that explanation is not yet fully understood). TTM is viewed as a logical (albeit pathological) response to internal and external forces.
- *Current internal and external forces have greater explanatory power than do historical events.* It is often tempting to attribute problem behaviors to historical events such as childhood abuse or other traumas. We do not doubt that childhood learning experiences can play a role in the etiology of TTM. However, these events in and of themselves cannot explain how and why the problem behavior started. Most people who have experienced traumas do not develop these kinds of problems, and in our clinical experience, most people with these problems deny a history of trauma. Therefore, early experiences can account for only a small portion of the variance in the development of TTM. We find it much more productive to focus on the here and now. Furthermore, this focus lends itself more readily to the development of active, specific interventions than does an historical focus.
- *The roots of TTM can be found in the person's physiological makeup, internal sensations, cognitions, and the consequences of the behavior itself; and these factors interact with one another.* The first part of this assumption suggests that individuals with TTM are different from the rest of the population in terms of their central or peripheral physiology, the kinds of internal sensations they experience, their cognitive appraisal of events, the kinds of rewards obtained by the problem behavior, or a combination of these factors. These differences may predispose the person to develop TTM, or they may develop over time as the problem becomes more deeply entrenched. The second part of the assumption reminds us that no single factor can be examined in isolation. To understand why a person finds hair pulling rewarding, for example, we must strive to understand also the internal and external pressures that triggered the behavior in the first place, as well as the physiological differences that might lead the person to find it rewarding.

Our model of TTM starts, as do other models, with a biological vulnerability of some kind; the implication here is that without this vulnerability, body-focused habits are less likely to blossom into full-blown impulse control disorders. This biological vulnerability may be manifest in the form of altered pain sensitivity, increased perception of negative internal states, or increased drive to engage in repetitive behavior. Negative internal states, as well as discriminative internal and external cues that have become associated with the behavior, trigger the onset of the problem behavior, perhaps through powerful internal urges to perform the behavior. The behavior itself is then rewarded in one of two ways: by decreasing negative internal emotions or thoughts, or by eliciting positive feelings. The positive sensations elicited by the behavior may be linked in part to the altered pain sensitivity, and the repeated hair pulling or other BFRB may also alter pain sensitivity further. These rewards increase the probability that the behavior will occur again. Pulling, picking, and other BFRBs are often associated with long-term negative social and emotional consequences, but these are not sufficient to override the immediate gratification obtained via the problem behavior, so the behavior persists. Below, we discuss each aspect of the model in detail.

Biological Vulnerability. Although biological predisposition cannot fully explain the onset of TTM, our model posits that certain biological factors "set the stage" for the onset of these disorders and hence increase the probability that an individual will develop such disorders. One such factor may be genetic: Familial research suggests that TTM and other BFBBs are associated with increased rates of OCD or other excessive habits among first-degree relatives (Bienvenu et al., 2000; King, Scahill et al., 1995; Lenane et al., 1992). This finding is consistent with the notion of a genetic basis for a spectrum of excessive grooming behaviors that includes TTM. Some authors have noted a similarity between TTM and excessive fixed action patterns of grooming seen in animals (Demaret, 1973; Swedo & Rapoport, 1991). Dogs and birds, for example, may evidence conditions known as acral lick dermatitis and feather picking disorder, respectively; interestingly, these conditions respond to serotonergic medications and/or naltrexone (Rapoport, Ryland, & Kriete, 1992; White, 1990; Wynchank & Berk, 1998), and early evidence suggests that behavior modification can also be effective (Bordnick, Thyer, & Ritchie, 1994; Eckstein & Hart, 1996; Jenkins, 2001). Rhesus monkeys often engage in hair pulling and eating when placed in a stressful, captive environment (Reinhardt, Reinhardt, & Houser, 1986). However, the hair pulling is largely other-directed rather than self-directed, and tends to follow social dominance lines (i.e., the more dominant monkey pulls the hair of less dominant monkeys); thus, the link to TTM is unclear.

Other evidence for a biological predisposition for TTM comes from neuroimaging research. For example, TTM patients exhibit hyperactivity in the left cerebellum and right superior parietal lobe (Swedo et al., 1991), as well as possible structural abnormalities in the left putamen (O'Sullivan et al., 1997), left inferior frontal gyrus, and right cuneal cortex (Grachev, 1997), although not all studies have identified differences between TTM patients and healthy controls (Stein, Coetzer, Lee, Davids, & Bouwer, 1997). Hyperactivity in frontal regions seems to decrease following pharmacological treatment (Stein et al., 2002). It is unknown whether behavioral treatment will also result in alterations in brain function, although such results have been reported in OCD (Baxter et al., 1992). It is also important to note that the neuroimaging findings are correlational; i.e., they only indicate an association between TTM and alterations in brain function, but do not necessarily imply causality. Studies of OCD, for example, have shown that when healthy participants are asked to think about obsessive topics, brain function is altered in ways that are similar in some ways to that of OCD patients (Cottraux et al., 1996). Thus, without longitudinal research, it cannot be determined whether preexisting brain abnormalities cause TTM, or whether engaging in hair pulling leads to alterations in brain function.

Neuropsychological studies are also consistent with alterations in brain functioning, although as with neuroimaging results, alternative explanations are also possible. TTM patients have been shown to make errors in spatial processing (Rettew, Cheslow, Rapoport, Leonard, & Lenane, 1991), divided attention (Stanley, Hannay, & Breckenridge, 1997), and nonverbal memory and executive functioning (Keuthen et al., 1996), although we note that in the latter study, Bonferroni correction for multiple comparisons would have made these differences nonsignificant. Studies such as these do not necessarily imply that preexisting brain abnormalities cause the symptoms of TTM; it is entirely possible that chronic TTM or its associated features lead to changes in brain structure or function, or that both TTM and the brain abnormalities are caused by a third, as yet unknown, variable.

We also suspect that a nonspecific biological vulnerability is manifested in difficulty tolerating discomfort. That is, individuals who feel a need to control or eliminate their uncomfortable emotions or sensations might be at greater risk to develop TTM and perhaps other disorders as well. This notion of "experiential avoidance" has been forwarded as a vulnerability factor for general psychopathology by Hayes and colleagues (e.g., Hayes, Strosahl, & Wilson, 1999), and intolerance of aversive states has been noted in anxiety disorders (Ladouceur, Gosselin, & Dugas, 2000; Reiss, Peterson, Gursky, & McNally, 1986; Tolin, Abramowitz, Brigidi, & Foa, 2003). A preliminary investigation of experiential avoidance in TTM suggested that a tendency to avoid unpleasant emotions was related to severity of hair-pulling urges (Begotka, Woods, & Wetterneck, 2003). However, the relationship, while significant, was relatively weak. This may relate to the fact that the investigators used a questionnaire that assessed primarily anxiety- and depression-related avoidance, rather than an avoidance of physiological arousal or other sensations that may be more directly applicable to TTM. This study also did not use a nonclinical control group; thus, range restriction may have been a factor. Clearly more research is needed to investigate the relationship between experiential avoidance and hair pulling and, more broadly, to examine whether experiential avoidance is related to biological factors and whether it represents a global diathesis for the development of maladaptive behaviors.

Altered Pain Sensitivity. Our working model also suggests that TMM/BFRBs are associated with alterations in the perception of pain. Individuals with TTM often report that hair-pulling is not painful (Christenson, MacKenzie et al., 1991; Sanderson & Hall-Smith, 1970). In fact, in many cases they report that it feels good or pleasurable (Stanley et al., 1992). Recently, we (Meunier, Tolin, & Franklin, 2005) surveyed children and adolescents with TTM about what it feels like to pull hair. Participants made significantly higher endorsements of the statements "It feels good" and "It makes me feel satisfied" than they did the statement "It hurts." One study of young children with short pulling histories also found low ratings of pain, suggesting that individuals with TTM may have a pre-existing alteration in pain sensitivity (Chang, Lee, Chiang, & Lu, 1991); this alteration may become even more pronounced with repeated pulling.

Thus, it is possible that alterations in pain sensitivity influence the reinforcing quality of pulling behavior. One possible mechanism for such alterations is upregulation of the endogenous opioid system; a recent challenge task supported this hypothesis in skin picking, but not TTM (Frecska & Arato, 2002), although some evidence suggests that pulling may decrease with administration of opiate receptor antagonists (Carrion, 1995; Christenson, Crow, & MacKenzie, 1994). Intriguingly, dogs with acral lick dermatitis (a potential animal model of TTM) show reductions in evoked sensory nerve action potentials (van Nes, 1986), possibly suggesting decreased pain sensitivity. However, TTM patients do not appear to show reduced pain in non-pulling areas such as the fingertips (Christenson et al., 1994). It may be that pain sensations are not globally altered in TTM, but rather are diminished only at the sites of pulling. This may result from habituation of the pain response caused by repeated pulling over time. There is a rich behavioral literature on *conditional analgesia*, in which stimuli that have been repeatedly associated with pain can eventually elicit an analgesic response, possibly mediated by endogenous opioids (see Faneslow, 1991, for a review). Thus, the act of repeated pulling or picking itself may eventually make pulling or picking less painful, as pre-pulling/picking stimuli (e.g., sitting in front of the television, or running fingers through hair) trigger a pre-emptive analgesic response. In our survey of children and adolescents with TTM (Meunier, Tolin, & Franklin, 2005), we asked children to describe how it felt to pull hair recently, as well as how it felt the first time they remember pulling hair. Ratings of the item "it felt good" did not differ between the two time points; however, ratings of the item "it hurt" were high for the first pull and significantly lower for the recent pull. At the first pull, participants strongly endorsed both items, suggesting that the first pull was associated with a mix of pleasure and pain. Over time, the pain sensation decreased, leaving the pleasure sensation unchecked, thus setting the stage for positive reinforcement. These ratings, relying on the subjective recall of children, must be considered tentative; ultimately, this issue must be addressed with longitudinal research.

For those patients who do experience pulling-related pain, the pain itself may be reinforcing by distracting the individual from negative emotional or physiological states (Christenson & Mansueto, 1999). Referring again to our survey of young people with TTM, we found that participants indicated that pulling made them feel calmer and less bored, and made them "zone out." Thus, even when pulling, picking, etc. are associated with pain, the behavior may still be reinforced by facilitating avoidance of more aversive internal states (Herrnstein, 1969). In the words of one of our patients, "I'd rather feel pain than anxiety."

Behavioral Triggers. Over time, after repeated pulling episodes, the problem behavior becomes associated with a variety of internal and external cues through classical conditioning (Azrin & Nunn, 1973; Mansueto et al., 1997). In the same way that one's mouth might begin to water when one enters a bakery, a person with TTM may start to experience urges to pull when he/she is in a place, doing an activity, or experiencing a sensation that has become associated with pulling. Being in this situation increases the likelihood of the behavior, which in turn strengthens the association. In this manner, a vicious cycle is born in which each instance of the behavior increases the likelihood of the next. In our model, we describe two forms of behavioral triggers: negative internal states and discriminative external cues.

Evidence for the association between negative internal states and TTM comes from descriptive research showing that these behaviors commonly follow a number of aversive states that might generally be classified as "dysregulated arousal." Thus, a person who is hyperaroused (e.g., is experiencing anger, stress, agitation, worry) or hypoaroused (e.g., is bored, or tired) is at increased risk for pulling, picking, etc. (Christenson, Ristvedt, & MacKenzie, 1993). In studies of TTM, researchers have found that hyperarousal triggers may include included negative emotions (e.g., feeling angry, hurt, anxious, or depressed) as well as situations associated with negative self-evaluation (e.g., weighing yourself, interpersonal conflicts). Hypoarousal triggers, on the other hand, may include situations associated with fatigue (e.g., lack of sleep), sedentary activity (e.g., reading, television), or feelings of boredom or apathy (Christenson et al., 1993; Simeon et al., 1997). Physical sensations have also been identified as arousal cues for hair pulling. For example, a substantial minority of TTM patients reported skin sensitivity (25%), itching (23%), irritation (16%), pressure (14%), and burning sensations (5%) as preceding pulling episodes (Mansueto, 1990).

Cognitive components are also involved at least to some extent in conceptualizing TTM, in that cognitions may serve as cues and consequences to the behavioral sequence. In some cases negative cognitions about the habit itself, such as fear of negative evaluation, may also play a role in the perpetuation of the behavior, as these cognitions result in increased negative emotion which in turn may increase urges to pull. Additionally, patients sometimes worry that the urges to engage in the behavior will never go away or will get stronger until the behavior is performed, despite their being able to provide ample evidence to the contrary from their own experience with urges. Beliefs in the positive effects of the behavior (e.g., "hair pulling will make me feel better") or facilitative thoughts (e.g., "I'll just pull one") may also cue pulling episodes (Gluhoski, 1995).

Another category of potential TTM triggers is contextual cues, which may not have originally been associated with pulling or pulling-related feelings or sensations, but by the process of associative conditioning have become linked with these factors through repetitive episodes or pulling. Common contextual cues for hair pulling include visual signs that hair is misshapen or unattractive (e.g., asymmetrical hair, gray hair), tactile sensations (e.g., feeling a coarse hair), places or activities where pulling has occurred in the past (e.g., bathroom, bed, watching television), being alone, or the presence of pulling implements (e.g., tweezers). Both arousal and contextual cues may be either associated with pulling directly or through the mediation of a hair pulling "urge". Over time, hair-pulling urges that are reinforced by pulling lead to stronger urges to pull, which perpetuates the behavioral cycle.

Reinforcement. As described earlier, pulling is often preceded by negative internal states such as unpleasant emotions, aversive physiological sensations, or dysregulated arousal. Pulling, in turn, appears to result in a decrease of these states. In retrospective reports, TTM patients report that pulling leads to reduced feelings of tension, boredom, and anxiety (Diefenbach, Tolin, Meunier et al., 2005), while nonclinical hair pullers also report reductions in sadness and anger (Stanley, Borden, Mouton, & Breckenridge, 1995). In these cases, hair-pulling is negatively reinforced and is thus functionally somewhat similar to the compulsive behaviors seen in OCD (Tolin & Foa, 2001). However, to the extent that hair-pulling evokes pleasurable sensations (Meunier, Tolin, & Franklin, 2005; Stanley et al., 1992), the pulling habit may also be strengthened via *positive* reinforcement (Azrin & Nunn, 1973; Mansueto et al., 1997; Meunier, Tolin, Diefenbach et al., 2005). Pleasure may be obtained not only through pulling, but also through associated behaviors such as playing with or inspecting the hair, oral stimulation, or trichophagia (Christenson & Mansueto, 1999; Rapp, Miltenberger, Galensky, Ellingson, & Long, 1999). Thus, pulling may be maintained by either negative or positive reinforcement. Our clinical observations suggest that some TTM patients may experience one or the other form of reinforcement, or different kinds of reinforcement may be active for the same person at different times. We propose that careful attention to the specific behavioral contingencies is critical in developing a functional analysis and planning therapeutic interventions for TTM.

Delayed Consequences of TTM. Although hair pulling is immediately reinforced via its consequent emotional or interoceptive changes, this behavior is also associated with longer-term negative consequences such as unwanted changes in physical appearance. Many persons with TTM experience baldness, scarring, and related problems, which often can only be concealed with substantial effort, if at all. The use of wigs or special make-up can be costly, time consuming, and uncomfortable. Patients also experience negative emotional consequences of their behavior such as guilt, sadness, and anger (Diefenbach, Mouton-Odum, & Stanley, 2002; Diefenbach, Tolin, Meunier et al., 2005), negative self-evaluation, frustrations with being out of control of pulling, and low self esteem (Casati, Toner, & Yu, 2000; Diefenbach, Tolin, Hannan et al., 2005; Soriano et al., 1996; Stemberger et al., 2000). TTM can also lead to negative social consequences.

In an experimental study, adolescents viewing videotapes of individuals pulling hair rated the hair-pullers as lower in social acceptability than they did those who were not pulling hair (Boudjouk, Woods, Miltenberger, & Long, 2000). Consequently, hair pullers have reported interpersonal conflicts, social isolation, and loneliness (Casati et al., 2000; Stemberger et al., 2000). Why, then, do these negative consequences not extinguish the problem behavior? We suspect that, as with many maladaptive behaviors (e.g., smoking, overeating) the short-term reinforcement value often overpowers the delayed aversive consequences. In fact, the longer-term consequences may even serve to escalate the pulling cycle by providing a new behavioral cue (e.g., negative self-evaluative thoughts, negative affect) that can prompt additional pulling episodes.

COMMUNICATING THE MODEL TO PATIENTS

Patients vary in terms of the degree of theoretical information that they need or want. Some patients, even many adolescents, are eager to learn everything they can about their disorder, and will readily engage in high-level discussions about biological and behavioral factors in TTM. Other patients prefer a "bare bones" discussion and want to get right to the interventions. We recommend, however, that all patients receive at least minimal information about TTM and the biopsychosocial model. A well-informed patient can be a valuable ally as treatment progresses: in the early stages, the patient who has a clear understanding of the function of their hair pulling can help generate ideas for treatment intervention. In later stages of treatment, as the patient becomes more independent, they can use their knowledge of TTM to effectively improvise new ways of gaining control. We present some examples of this kind of psychoeducation in Chapter 6.

In many cases, the diagram in Figure 1 can be used as a vehicle for discussing our current understanding of TTM. Although the diagram in total is a bit dense for many patients, our experience has been that if the therapist goes through each part of the model slowly, eliciting questions along the way, many patients report that they find it helpful to see TTM "mapped out." Some of the questions that the therapist is likely to encounter are described in Chapter 6. It is important to respond accurately and honestly to patients' questions; this often means discussing current knowledge of TTM as well as the limitations of what is known. We have been pleasantly surprised to find that our patients, young and old, usually do not mind when we do not have all the answers. Regardless of the question, effective therapists frame their answers using language that is appropriate to age and developmental status, using examples and metaphors that the patient can understand.

CHAPTER 3

WHAT IT IS AND WHAT IT ISN'T:

Diagnostics, Differential Diagnosis, and Review of Clinical Measures

DIAGNOSTICS

We reviewed the DSM-IV-TR definition of TTM in Chapter 1 and return to it now to discuss more specifically how to evaluate TTM patients in accordance with DSM criteria. We know from previous studies that some patients who endorse hair pulling and resultant alopecia do not meet full DSM-IV-TR criteria (specifically the requirement of increasing tension and relief), and that this tendency might be more evident with younger patients for developmental reasons. We discuss these issues at length below.

We endeavored in this section to consider the assessment burden carefully, given that most of the readers of this volume are likely to be working in clinical settings where market forces limit the amount of time that can be spent on diagnostics. Regardless of setting, it is our belief that a comprehensive assessment of TTM should include evaluation of the DSM-IV-TR criteria as well as examination of the more common comorbid psychiatric diagnoses that are described below. The clinical data that we have analyzed thus far in our pediatric TTM study has suggested that those presenting to participate in our clinical trials of CBT thus far have had relatively low rates of comorbid psychopathology (Franklin, Keuthen et al., 2002; Tolin et al., 2006); compared to adult samples (Christenson et al., 1992; Christenson, MacKenzie et al., 1991; Diefenbach, Tolin, Hannan, Maltby, & Crocetto, in press). It is important to screen for comorbid conditions since the failure to detect co-occurring disorders prior to initiating CBT may later prove costly with respect to treatment compliance and, ultimately, outcome.

TTM DIAGNOSIS

TTM is not surveyed on the major semi-structured interview measures for adults [e.g., Structured Diagnostic Interview for DSM-IV (SCID; First, Spitzer, Gibbon, & Williams, 1995)] and children [e.g., Schedule for Affective Disorders and Schizophrenia for School-age Children (K-SADS; Ambrosini, 2000)], which might be one practical reason that the condition is understudied; it was also not screened for recent psychiatric epidemiology studies (e.g., National Comorbidity Survey and its replication), either because of the lack of a reliable and valid measure at the time those studies were developed, or perhaps because of the perception at the that TTM is an extremely rare disorder (see Chapter 1 for a discussion of the estimated prevalence of TTM). In our work with both adults and younger patients, we have adapted Rothbaum and Ninan's (1994) Trichotillomania Diagnostic Interview (TDI) to survey DSM-IV-TR criteria during initial interviews with prospective TTM clinical patients or clinical research participants. Formal study of the psychometric properties of the DSM-IV-TR version of the TDI adapted for use with children and adolescents is underway in our research group; we are not aware of such studies with adults.

Following the format of the SCID with other psychiatric disorders, the TDI yields scores on each of the DSM-IV-TR criteria A through D, and also includes a comprehensive checklist of possible pulling sites. Each criterion is ranked as either absent (1), subthreshold (2), or threshold/true (3). Because the TDI was developed using DSM III-R criteria, however, supplemental questions are needed to assess DSM-IV-TR Criterion B (increasing tension) and Criterion E (clinically significant distress/functional impairment) (see Appendix). Ratings of "3" on each item yield a DSM-IV-TR diagnosis of TTM. However, as we discussed above, some individuals who present for assessment and treatment of chronic and clinically significant hair pulling that has resulted in noticeable alopecia do not endorse Criteria B or C, which means that a formal diagnosis of TTM is not technically warranted. Nevertheless, we know of no compelling research suggesting that these individuals differ in clinically important ways from those who meet the full criteria, and we tend in our clinical practice to proceed accordingly.

In terms of when and how to conduct the TDI interview clinically, we generally follow the format suggested by Rothbaum, Opdyke, and Keuthen (1999), who advocate for an initial open clinical interview that will allow for the establishment of rapport and will provide the patient an opportunity to tell the story of their hair pulling. We tend to view this initial interview as a wonderful opportunity for psychoeducation, and tailor the discussion to the particular patient's previous experience with psychotherapy, knowledge of TTM and its treatment, etc. Once we have learned a bit about the patient's history and about their history with TTM, we then move to the evaluation of DSM-IV-TR criteria via the TDI, and preface that interview with a general discussion about TTM and "what some people with trich have reported about their pulling." We also emphasize to our patients that they are the experts in their particular problems and that we are experts in helping people to think about and solve such problems, and that effective treatment will require both kinds of expertise. This approach underscores the prevailing message that we wish to convey in the initial assessment and throughout the treatment: TTM is a known entity that we have encountered frequently in our clinical practice; the heterogeneity of TTM reported by others with the disorder suggests that not all TTM is the same and therefore each individual patient has much to teach us; and it is imperative to discuss the details of TTM openly so that the clinician will be in the best possible position to be helpful to the patient. We also wish to convey to the patient that we admire their courage in coming forward to seek assistance with TTM, and that we recognize the inherent difficulty in discussing TTM with other people.

Assessing Criterion A can be relatively straightforward if the patient is obviously bald, wearing a wig, or has missing eyebrows or eyelashes, so we caution clinicians not to simply read the question as if he/she is not privy to this information already. In the spirit of the matter-of-fact frankness we wish to convey in the treatment setting, we ask the patient if we can do a visual inspection of the resultant bald areas on the scalp, eyelashes, or eyebrows, and respect the patient's response to our request. If the pulling sites listed on the TDI checklist are not readily evident upon visual inspection or if the patient has gone to considerable lengths to disguise the damage (e.g., penciling in eyebrows, false eyelashes), we will ask them to describe the pulling site and what percentage of hair has been removed via pulling.

We move next to Criterion B, which involves "an increasing sense of tension immediately before pulling out the hair or when attempting to resist the behavior." For the many TTM patients who do experience this tension, the answer to this question comes readily, whereas for others further probing is needed before we can conclude with confidence that there is no pre-pulling tension evident. We ask them to recall their affective and physical states prior to their last pulling episode to give the discussion more context, establish if this last episode was at least somewhat representative of most of their pulling episodes, ask they were feeling "keyed up" or as if they had a physical urge to itch that required scratching, which is another way that patients may describe this pre-pulling physical sensation. Those whose pulling is truly automatic may still not endorse Criterion B, which is when we switch to asking about the last time they were aware that they had been pulling and had made an attempt to stop, then we ask about affective and physical states again as before. Younger patients may have difficulty introspecting about their internal states or difficulty describing such states, which requires some non-verbal demonstrations of the experience of tension, which we usually do by balling up our fists, making an uncomfortable face, and shifting uncomfortably in our seat, while saying, "Do you feel kind of like this right before you pull?" For some children this demonstration helps them grasp the concept better and will allow for a more valid answer.

If the patient responds that the pulling was not driven by tension but instead was a response to a thought that had to be neutralized or (less frequently) was in response to a voice commanding them to do so, we begin to consider some of the differential diagnoses described below. On rare occasions, we encounter patients who tell us that they were pulling because they were feeling empty or feeling nothing and wanted to feel pain rather than emptiness; with these patients we tend to probe further into other self-destructive behaviors (e.g., cutting, burning) as the pulling in such cases may be serving a very different affective function than it does in the vast majority of patients with TTM. In general we do not view typical TTM as a form of "self-mutilation;" we dismiss psychoanalytic conceptualizations of the disorder that lack any empirical foundation, and are clear to convey this to our patients, too many of whom have been exposed at some point to these views.

Criterion C often requires significant probing for the minority of patients who do not immediately describe the pulling as producing pleasure, satisfaction, or relief. It is important to preface this question with an empathic statement such as, "I can see from what you've described that trich is causing lots of problems in your life, and these problems led you to come see me today. However, the questions I'm about to ask have to do with how you feel right as you are engaging in the pulling." With this statement we hope to create an atmosphere in which patients will be comfortable sharing with us that pulling is pleasurable in some way – this is often a source of shame, and therefore it is important to attempt to overcome this barrier to disclosure. Before asking in more detail about affective responses to pulling, we will say, "When describing the feelings they experience right as they are pulling, lots of folks with trich report that they found it pleasurable or satisfying in some way, or like it was a relief – sort of how you feel after you scratch an itch that's been bothering you. Do you feel any of these kinds of things while you pull?" We recommend a similar approach with children and adolescents, many of whom are even more reluctant to report honestly about pleasure in response to pulling because of the obvious negative impact the TTM is having on their families. Sometimes the younger children will respond, "I don't know," when asked if pulling felt good in some way as they were doing it, but our clinical experience leads us to probe a bit further at that point, especially if a child that had been making eye contact with the therapist now averts their gaze as they respond to this question. A simple statement such as, "I've also met lots of kids with trich who have trouble answering that question, because they're afraid to say that a behavior that's causing so much trouble for them and their families actually feels good when they are doing it." Again, young children have developmentally appropriate difficulty with introspection and with describing affective states, so there is an increased chance that within this age group there will be no clear answer to this question.

Criterion D requires that TTM is not better accounted for by another mental disorder and is not due to a general medical condition. For Criterion D it is important to ask specifically about recent medical history, initiation of and/or changes in medication regimen, history of skin problems such as eczema, other dermatological problems, and other such possible explanations for alopecia such as alopecia areata, which is distinguished from TTM by the presence of inflammation (DSM-IV, pp. 619). Some other psychiatric conditions can occasionally be associated with hair pulling, and these are discussed in detail below in the section on differential diagnosis.

Criterion E, that the disturbance causes clinically significant distress or impairment in role functioning is virtually standard in DSM-IV-TR. In the clinic we rarely have difficulty establishing this for our adult patients (see Table 1). Most of the children and adolescents that we see also describe restricted activities, embarrassment and shame, social avoidance, and a host of problems that impact their functioning. However, we do occasionally see young children whose pulling appears to be only minimally disturbing to them, even though it is extremely difficult on their parents. Here psychoeducation can be useful, in that many parents fear for the child's future ability to make friends, succeed in school, and live a happy life, and they may also harbor concerns that their own parenting "caused" the TTM. We try to reassure parents that there is no single cause of TTM, and that there is really very little that they may have done or said that probably made the child begin and continue pulling. We also try to assist parents in recognizing that if the child appears to be functioning very well in school now, has friends, and appears to be happy and unconcerned about the TTM, their motivation to change this behavior now will likely affect CBT compliance and, by extension, outcome. We encourage families whose children do not appear to be at all upset about TTM to think about whether this is the right time to initiate CBT, as we already see a risk factor for CBT non-compliance and attenuated outcome. Of course with young children we can and often do add in contingency management strategies to stimulate motivation to comply with CBT methods, as many children do not fully appreciate the long-term implications of behavior and are more responsive to proximal rewards. However, when children are not at all bothered by their pulling or its consequences, wonder why they are in the therapist's office at all, and are demonstrably unable or unwilling to engage in a treatment process that will require substantial effort on their part to reduce a behavior that they do not see as problematic, the best strategy may be to delay treatment initiation until such time as the child's view changes. Prochaska and DiClemente have spoken eloquently about the process of behavior change for a wide variety of problematic behaviors, and perhaps one of the most important contributions of their seminal work is the observation that forcing very active interventions upon people who are not in the right "stage of change" can do more harm than good (for a review see Prochaska, DiClemente, & Norcross, 1992).

OTHER PSYCHIATRIC DIAGNOSES

The literature on psychiatric comorbidity in adults and, perhaps to a lesser extent, children and adolescents, suggests that it is important to survey routinely for the more commonly co-occurring conditions. In the clinical research context this is usually done via semi-structured clinical interview, the majority of which take two to three hours to complete. Such an exhaustive assessment may not be feasible in most clinical practice settings, yet the importance of gathering clinically relevant information about common comorbidities remains. Interviews such as the MINI or the KID-MINI (Sheehan et al., 1998) may bridge this gap in that they include brief screening questions for most of the major psychiatric illnesses but do not require the same amount of time to complete; less optimally, such interviews could be used when data from the patient's history or in their initial presentation for TTM treatment arouses suspicion that other disorders of relevance may also be present. Depression has been reported to be the most common of the co-occurring disorders and accordingly some measure of depression would seem to be required, regardless of whether the MINI or KID-MINI is also employed. Substance abuse also appears to be a common co-occurring condition, and should also be screened for routinely. In the section on measures below we describe some of the more commonly used measures for these purposes and also include a listing of measures that can be used to screen for other conditions that may co-occur with TTM (e.g., anxiety disorders). It is also important to establish the timing of and the primacy of any co-occurring disorders that are uncovered upon screening, since this information will likely influence treatment planning. For example, treatment for the patient who reports that their depression preceded pulling and whose pulling is strongly influenced by mood problems would likely be treated quite differently from a patient whose depression clearly followed the onset of TTM, which seems to have developed in reaction to the functional impairment and social avoidance associated with his/her hair pulling.

DIFFERENTIAL DIAGNOSIS

Not all hair pulling necessarily falls under the diagnostic umbrella of TTM, and it is important to consider those psychiatric conditions that may involve hair pulling behavior but are not best explained under the biopsychosocial model we presented in Chapter 2, which was created to be inclusive yet not all-encompassing.

Sometimes these diagnostic debates have more academic than clinical relevance, and the final diagnosis will not influence the delivery of treatment, but this is not the case for the conditions we describe below. In our view it is important to distinguish these from TTM as we conceptualized it above, and to encourage patients who are diagnosed with these conditions to seek alternative treatment.

OBSESSIVE-COMPULSIVE DISORDER

TTM involves chronic behavioral repetition, and as such shares some formal similarity with OCD. Indeed, the relationship between OCD, TTM, and other conditions involving problematic repetitive behaviors has been conceptualized as representing a continuum that is now often referred to as the "OC Spectrum" (for a comprehensive review see Hollander, 1993). TTM does possess some features that allow it to be distinguished from OCD, such as its generally being maintained by positive rather than negative reinforcement (Stanley et al., 1992), the absence of intrusive, repetitive thoughts that precede the behavior (Stanley & Mouton, 1996; Stanley et al., 1993; Stanley et al., 1992), and the tendency toward a single compulsive behavior in TTM patients as opposed to multiple types of rituals in individuals with OCD (Stanley et al., 1992). One of our patients reported that she pulled her hair out whenever she had an intrusive image of harm befalling a loved one, and that she felt a reduction in her obsessional distress when the hair had been extracted. Upon further inquiry it also became evident that she engaged in other repetitive behaviors such as moving objects from one spot to another (e.g., coffee cup across the desk) that served this same neutralizing function. She denied that the hair pulling itself was pleasurable or satisfying in any way (in fact she found it painful), but nevertheless she did it in order to decrease her distress and to reduce the likelihood that something catastrophic would happen to someone she cared about. Together these observations led us to believe that a diagnosis of OCD rather than TTM was warranted and that, unlike in CBT for TTM, a significant amount of imaginal exposure to the feared disasters would be needed in order to reduce her symptoms (for a review of OCD treatment strategies see Franklin & Foa, 2002). We recommend that readers make this same distinction in their own work, and either treat such patients for OCD using empirically validated techniques or, if this is not an area of expertise, refer to a specialist who treats OCD.

PSYCHOTIC DISORDERS

DSM-IV-TR clearly specifies that hair pulling in response to a delusion or hallucination of any kind should not be considered under the definition of TTM, but rather grouped with psychotic disorders. We have rarely encountered this in our specialty clinics, but it is important to query the patient's understanding of what leads to pulling. The questions about what leads to pulling, which are usually asked when surveying for Criterion B, should be asked carefully so as to elicit sufficient information to rule out the possibility of an underlying psychotic disorder. Sometimes patients give somewhat unusual answers to these questions (e.g., "My hands have a mind of their own;" "It's like it's a punishment from God"), and it is important to query further to determine if these statements are meant metaphorically. If not, or if the patient's answers further suggest the possibility of thought disorder (e.g., "I pull out the hairs to get the demons out of my body"), then it is imperative to conduct a more comprehensive evaluation for other symptoms of psychotic disorder rather than to simply proceed with the TTM evaluation. The psychotic disorder itself clearly takes precedence in this circumstance, and should be the target of the assessment; referral to relevant clinical services is also essential. The patient's developmental and treatment history as well as their cultural background may prove helpful in making this evaluation: One of our patients said that she was pulling because the devil made her, but her explanation was supported in full by her deeply religious family, who viewed the TTM symptoms as a struggle against evil and thought their daughter's symptoms were insulting to God. In this case, we did not diagnose a psychotic disorder and proceeded with the TTM interview. Relatedly, members of several ethnic and cultural minority groups frequently describe symptoms in a manner that some ethnic majority interviewers may regard as psychotic (e.g., culturally-held beliefs in spiritualism). Thus, interviewers must be extra sensitive to the possibility of misdiagnosing psychotic disorders when working cross-culturally.

BODY DYSMORPHIC DISORDER

Some years ago we assessed a woman in an OCD outpatient clinic whose symptoms focused primarily on the appearance of her hair, which she viewed as "ugly," "uncontrollable," and "offensive." Body image dissatisfaction is unfortunately all too common generally in the United States, particularly among women, and sometimes this self-critical tendency extends to the hair. In this case, however, the patient was spending up to nine hours per day checking, cutting, and pulling the hairs she deemed most offensive. There was a sufficient amount of pulling amongst these other compulsive rituals to suggest that a secondary diagnosis of TTM might be warranted, but here the DSM system precludes the TTM diagnosis since the hair pulling is subsumed under the BDD diagnosis. Similarly, dissatisfaction with appearance is very commonly reported in TTM, but the secondary diagnosis of BDD is precluded in part because the resultant distress is accounted for in TTM Criterion E and because the perceived defect usually neither imagined nor greatly exaggerated. If other body image dissatisfaction is present then a diagnosis of comorbid BDD may be appropriate, and needs to be considered in the clinical context of focused treatment on TTM.

BORDERLINE PERSONALITY DISORDER

We mentioned earlier that we sometimes encounter patients whose pulling behavior appears to be prompted by chronic feelings of emptiness or is an attempt to feel pain rather than feeling nothing. We mentioned also that most TTM patients experience pulling as pleasurable rather than painful, although there are exceptions. Nevertheless, this kind of initial explanation for pulling prompts us to ask about other features of borderline personality disorder (BPD), such as a pattern of unstable interpersonal relationships, extreme response to real or imagined abandonment, identity disturbance, impulsivity, recurrent suicidal behavior, gestures, or threats, or other forms of self-harm such as cutting or burning. In and of itself, TTM should not be considered sufficient for a diagnosis of comorbid BPD, regardless of the patient's affective response to pulling. As with patients with possible psychotic disorder, however, if it does become evident that BPD is the primary diagnosis it is important to conduct a thorough evaluation and provide appropriate clinical referrals if the assessing clinician is not well versed in BPD or in dialectical behavior therapy (DBT; Linehan, 1993), which is developing an evidence base as an efficacious treatment for reducing parasuicidal behaviors in BPD (e.g., Westen, 2000).

REVIEW OF CLINICAL MEASURES

We recommend that whenever possible clinicians make use of the measures that are already available in the literature as opposed to creating their own, since this will improve standardization and also facilitate data collection and interpretation. We view data collection as an essential element of any CBT program, and in our section on implementing treatment we will describe how we make use of data in the clinical context. We also recognize that time constraints and financial pressures preclude the kind of comprehensive data collection methods that are used in clinical trials, and have structured our recommendations accordingly. The interested reader is referred to previous reviews (Diefenbach, Tolin, Crocetto, Maltby, & Hannan, 2005; Rothbaum et al., 1999; Stanley, Breckenridge, Snyder, & Novy, 1999) for comprehensive discussions of all of the available TTM measures and their intended uses.

DIAGNOSTIC INTERVIEWS

As discussed above, a modified version of Rothbaum and Ninan's (1994) TDI should be used to evaluate whether patients meet DSM-IV-TR criteria for TTM (see appendix). Information gathered during this diagnostic interview may also prompt consideration of differential diagnoses, discussion of the patient's relevant medical history, and deliberation of whether TTM is sufficiently impairing to warrant clinical intervention. We also mentioned above that the wording of the TDI requires some modification for children and adolescents, and we have included the modification and some suggested prompts in the appendix as well. We also recommend that the clinician have the MINI or the KID-MINI (Sheehan et al., 1998) available for routine screening of common comorbid conditions if at all feasible; at the very least these instruments provide a structured set of follow-up questions if the clinician has evidence from an unstructured clinical interview suggesting the presence of depression or other disorders of relevance. These diagnostic measures can also be given again at the end of treatment to determine the effect of CBT on TTM and the comorbid conditions (if any), as this information will be important in guiding end-of-treatment recommendations.

TTM MEASURES

NIMH Trichotillomania Questionnaire (Swedo et al., 1989). Derived from the Yale-Brown Obsessive Compulsive Scale (Y-BOCS; Goodman, Price, Rasmussen, Mazure, Delgado et al., 1989; Goodman, Price, Rasmussen, Mazure, Fleischmann et al., 1989) and the Leyton Obsessional Inventory (LOI; Cooper, 1970), this semi-structured clinical interview consists of two clinician-rated scales: the NIMH Trichotillomania Severity Scale (NIMH-TSS) and the NIMH Trichotillomania Impairment Scale (NIMH-TIS). The NIMH-TSS consists of five questions related to the following aspects of trichotillomania: average time spent pulling, time spent pulling on the previous day, resistance to urges, resulting distress, and daily interference. NIMH-TSS scores range from 0–25. The NIMH-TIS is a clinician rating of patient impairment with scores ranging from 0–10; higher scores on both scales indicate greater severity/impairment. Psychometric data for the NIMH Trichotillomania Questionnaire are limited, but good inter-rater reliability has been reported in two small studies (Diefenbach et al., 2006; Swedo et al., 1989). The NIMH-TSS has been shown to be sensitive to changes in symptom severity and impairment following treatment (Lerner et al., 1998; Rothbaum, 1992; Swedo et al., 1989). Although much of its previous use has been with adults, it has also been used to measure TTM symptom severity in studies that included children and adolescents (Franklin, Keuthen et al., 2002; Lerner et al., 1998). The reliability and validity of the NIMH scales with younger samples is currently under investigation at our respective centers.

Self-Monitoring. Self-monitoring is a core element of the CBT approach that we espouse, and accordingly is discussed in detail in a subsequent chapter. For our purpose here in discussing outcome measurement, we will focus on the fact that we ask patients to write down the individual number of hairs pulled in all pulling episodes, which can then be translated into graphs for the patient and clinician to review in each session. Many of our younger patients are computer savvy and enjoy actually entering their own self-monitoring data into the Microsoft Powerpoint data charts that we keep for them on our computers (password protected and without their names, of course). These graphs become extremely useful over time in underscoring when progress is being made as well as identifying when there are upturns in pulling, and in helping patients to think about the reasons for these increases. Pulling site complicates the use of these data considerably, in that those who pull eyelashes and eyebrows may have a more episodic pattern and therefore progress may not be as easily captured using this method. We suggest having such patients rate the intensity of pulling urges as well, since this will allow a more stable measure of the persistence of TTM symptoms.

Alopecia Ratings. Assessment of TTM-related alopecia is fraught with both methodological and clinical difficulties, but it is important nevertheless to attempt. Subjective ratings of alopecia severity at each pulling site (e.g., scalp, eyelashes) can be made by patients and clinicians – we include in the appendix the rating scale that is being used by trained raters in our clinical research trials. In our research trials we have used repeated photographs of the pulling site(s) to document treatment progress; the suitability of such photographs in clinical practice should be considered carefully by both therapist and patient. The reliability and validity of such measures has not been the subject of much research to date, although one study found strong inter-rater reliability (Diefenbach et al., 2005). Other objective measures have been used in research settings such as measurement of hair density, weight and number of collected pulled hairs (for a review see Diefenbach, Reitman, & Williamson, 2000).

Clinically it may be difficult for patients to agree to let the clinician look carefully at, or photograph, their pulling sites. As with much of what we request in the context of CBT, we provide a clear rationale for the request, explain clearly how this information will be used, and provide feedback from our clinical experience about how some of our previous patients have found the record of hair growth over time be helpful to reminding them about the progress they have made in treatment.

Saving Pulled Hairs. Many of the same methodological and clinical issues we discussed above with respect to alopecia photographs are germane when it comes to asking patients to save pulled hairs. As discussed in detail in Chapter 7, we provide a clear rationale for the importance of the procedure, let patients who are reluctant know that they are not alone among our previous patients in having reservations about it, and tell them specifically that we will look at the saved hairs when we review self-monitoring materials and then discard the hairs in their presence.

Massachusetts General Hospital Hairpulling Scale (MGH-HPS; Keuthen et al., 1995; O'Sullivan et al., 1995). The MGH-HPS is a widely used self-report survey of the frequency, intensity, and control over hair pulling urges and behaviors and also evaluates associated distress. The psychometric properties of the scale are satisfactory (Diefenbach et al., 2005; Keuthen et al., 1995; O'Sullivan et al., 1995), and the instrument has been used in several outcome studies and found sensitive to treatment related changes. We recommend that the MGH-HPS be used at least before and after treatment to document treatment effects and to inform clinical decision-making. The same group of investigators have also developed self-report scales of skin-picking severity (Keuthen, Wilhelm et al., 2001) and associated impairment (Keuthen, Deckersbach et al., 2001) that are recommended for those patients with comorbid TTM and skin picking or for those with skin-picking alone.

Trichotillomania Scale for Children (TSC; Diefenbach, Tolin, Franklin, & Anderson, 2003). The TSC is a 15-item self-report questionnaire designed to assess several clinically relevant features of hair pulling behavior in children and adolescents. The TSC contains three subscales (severity, distress, impairment) comprised of five items each. Item response choices on the TSC range from 0–2 with higher numbers indicating more severe symptoms. The initial study of the TSC's psychometric properties (Diefenbach et al., 2003) was encouraging although the sample size was small; currently TSC data analyses are underway in our research group that will clarify the clinical utility of the TSC.

SCALES FOR COMMON COMORBIDITIES IN ADULTS

Depression Anxiety Stress Scales (DASS; Lovibond & Lovibond, 1995). The DASS is a 42-item self-report measure yielding three scales (depression, anxiety, and stress). A briefer version, the DASS-21, is also available. The DASS shows very good test-retest reliability and internal consistency, and the three scales appear to distinguish their respective constructs well (Antony, Bieling, Cox, Enns, & Swinson, 1998; Lovibond & Lovibond, 1995).

Sheehan Disability Scale (SDS; Leon, Shear, Portera, & Klerman, 1992). The SDS is a three-item self-report measure of work, social, and family impairment. Despite being a very short measure, the SDS shows high internal consistency reliability and strong construct validity, demonstrated by significantly different scores between individuals with and without psychiatric disorders (Leon, Olfson, Portera, Farber, & Sheehan, 1997). A significant relationship has been found between anxiety symptoms and impairment as measured by the SDS, signifying criterion-related validity (Leon et al., 1992). In addition, the SDS scores have been found to be sensitive to change over time. Although several broader and lengthier measures of impairment and quality of life disruption have been developed, there is little evidence that they outperform the much briefer SDS (Maltby, Diefenbach, Tolin, Crocetto, & Worhunsky, 2004).

SCALES FOR COMMON COMORBIDITIES IN CHILDREN AND ADOLESCENTS

Multidimensional Anxiety Scale for Children (MASC; March, Parker, Sullivan, Stallings, & Conners, 1997). This scale has four factors and six subfactors – physical anxiety (tense/restless, somatic/autonomic), harm avoidance (perfectionism, anxious coping), social anxiety (humiliation/rejection, performance), and separation anxiety. It is used in a variety of treatment outcome studies including the recently completed pediatric TTM RCT. The MASC has demonstrated excellent test-retest reliability and convergent/divergent validity (March et al., 1997), and takes approximately 10 minutes for the child to complete.

Children's Depression Inventory (CDI; Kovacs, 1985). This self-report scale inventories cognitive, affective, behavioral, and interpersonal symptoms of depression and has demonstrated adequate psychometric properties (Kovacs, 1985). The measure takes approximately 10 minutes for the child to complete, and is included in light of concerns about the relationship between TTM and depression. Here again we suggest that the CDI be given more frequently if the initial score is elevated (e.g., greater than 10).

CHAPTER 4

DOING THE DETECTIVE WORK:

Comprehensive Assessment of TTM

BEYOND DIAGNOSIS

This chapter picks up where Chapter 3 leaves off. We assume that the diagnosis of TTM/BFRB has already been established, as have any comorbid disorders. However, this information alone is not necessarily sufficient to develop an individualized treatment protocol. Establishing a diagnosis is a minimal criterion for treatment decision-making, but does not provide the necessary information to determine which specific interventions will help a given patient. For this task, a more fine-grained, comprehensive assessment is necessary. Thus, we consider assessment to be an integral part of treatment planning (e.g., tailoring specific interventions to match the patients needs), rather than a perfunctory step prior to treatment. The biopsychosocial model described in Chapter 2 can be used as an assessment guide during this step; the role of the comprehensive assessment is to flesh out some of the specific elements of the model. We will describe this process in detail below.

FUNCTIONAL ANALYSIS

Functional analysis is based on the premise that all behavior is influenced by its antecedents (events that tend to precede the behavior) and consequences (events that tend to follow the behavior). Antecedents to pulling/picking can be external (e.g., settings or activities that have become associated with pulling) or internal (e.g., emotions, thoughts, or internal sensations that trigger pulling). For the purpose of this assessment, "consequences" refers to immediate reinforcers for the behavior, both positive (e.g., obtaining pleasurable sensations) and negative (e.g., escaping unpleasant sensations). A clear understanding of the antecedents and consequences of pulling/picking behavior will often yield critical clues for treatment planning. It is particularly important to understand the *current* antecedents and consequences of the behavior, rather than only when the behavior first started. In many cases, the contingencies for the behavior can change over time, so that situations, feelings, etc., that were originally associated with pulling/picking are no longer associated, and previously unassociated antecedents and consequences have become associated with pulling/picking over time. For example, in a recent survey of children and adolescents with TTM, we found that sensations with pain tend to decrease over time, and that overall, pulling appears to become more pleasurable (Meunier, Tolin, & Franklin, 2005).

At first glance, it is easy to underestimate the challenge of gathering a good functional analysis. After all, asking the patient what happens before and after pulling/picking is not inherently difficult. However, establishing a probable causal relationship raises problems that are familiar to statisticians and researchers, but have substantial clinical relevance as well. It is not enough to note that pulling occurs often in a particular context. This does not establish the relationship and may lead the clinician down the wrong path. For example, pulling occurs often in the context of breathing, but this does not imply that breathing is a trigger for pulling, because the person (presumably) often breathes *without* pulling. Thus, functional analysis is best conceptualized as a two-by-two matrix:

		Pull?	
		Yes	No
Stimulus Present?	Yes		
	No		

For example, imagine that a patient has told us that she often pulls hair while watching TV. This is certainly helpful information. But before jumping to the conclusion that TV watching triggers her hair pulling, we want to determine the degree of association between watching TV and pulling. We ask the patient to estimate the percentage of time spent under each of these four conditions. The patient responds as follows:

		Pull?	
		Yes	No
Watching TV?	Yes	20%	30%
	No	40%	10%

In this case we can see that the patients initial statement—that she often pulls hair while watching TV—is true. However, we also see that this statement is probably true simply because she spends a lot of time (50% of her time, to be precise) watching TV. When watching TV, she spends more time *not* pulling (30%) than pulling (20%). We also see that she is more likely to pull when *not* watching TV (40%) than when watching TV (20%). Therefore, we would not consider TV watching to be strongly associated with pulling. Alternatively, imagine that the patient provides the following information:

		Pull?	
		Yes	No
Watching TV?	Yes	20%	5%
	No	10%	65%

In this case, we see that while watching TV, the patient is more likely to pull (20%) than not to pull (5%). We also see that when not watching TV, she is more likely not to pull (65%) than to pull (10%). This represents a clearer indication that TV watching may be functioning as a trigger for hair pulling. This situation, therefore, will be a target of specific interventions such as stimulus control (described in Chapter 8).

DETAILED INTERVIEW

A sample interview format is included in Appendix B. Note that the purpose of this interview is not to diagnose TTM or rule out comorbid disorders; it is assumed that these tasks have already been accomplished by this stage of the assessment. Rather, the goal is for the therapist and patient to develop a more thorough understanding of the functional context of the patients pulling behaviors. At the end of the interview is a "blank" copy of the TTM diagram from Chapter 2. As the therapist learns more about the patients pulling, he/she can write specific details into the diagram. We recommend giving patients a copy of this diagram, with their own information included. Many patients find it helpful and thought provoking to be able to refer to this diagram as they progress through treatment.

Early triggers. Antecedents can be thought of in terms of a chain of events that lead up to the pulling behavior. Presumably, the earlier the patient can intervene, the more likely it is that he/she will be able to refrain from the behavior. Therefore, asking about the earliest detectable antecedents is helpful. We often find it helpful to ask the patient to start at the point of pulling, and work backwards to the earliest antecedents they can identify. Possible early triggers include (but are certainly not limited to):

a. Setting: Where and when does the behavior take place? Are other people there?
b. Activities: What is the patient doing at the time?

c. Posture: How is the patient standing, sitting, or lying? In particular, where does he/she keep her hands?

d. Thoughts: What is the patient thinking about?

e. Emotions: How is the patient feeling?

f. Physiological sensations: What bodily sensations (e.g., muscular, gastrointestinal, cardiac, respiratory) is the patient feeling?

g. Arousal level: Is the patient feeling hyperaroused (e.g., hyper, tense, scattered) or hypoaroused (e.g., bored, tired, sleepy)?

h. Urges: Is the patient experiencing any urges to pull? If so, how are these urges experienced?

Different patients may describe very different early antecedents, and many patients will report different antecedents for different pulling episodes; therefore, it is important to gather this information across multiple episodes.

To illustrate how we gather this information, we will describe the functional assessment of two fictitious patients,[1] Claudia, a 17-year-old girl, and Howard, a 42-year-old man. We will begin with an investigation of Claudias early antecedents.

Therapist (T): Id like to get a better understanding of how your hair pulling goes. Lets start by talking about the place where it occurs. Where is the location in which you are most likely to pull?

Claudia (C): Well, I pull in a lot of different places but Id say that one place where I pull a lot is when Im studying for class after dinner.

T: When youre studying for class after dinner. Okay, thats helpful for me to know. Where do you usually study?

C: Mostly in my room.

T: Where in your room? Do you sit at a desk, or sit in bed?

C: I sit at a desk.

T: Okay, so you pull a lot when youre studying in your room at your desk. Is the door open or closed?

C: I always keep my door closed when Im studying. My brothers make so much noise during the evening that its hard for me to concentrate.

T: Gotcha. I know how hard it can be to try to study when someone is making a lot of noise! Now, when you sit at your desk, how do you sit? Can you show me?

---

[1] As with all of our patient examples throughout this book, the transcripts are not verbatim; rather, they represent a composite of many clinical experiences we have had with TTM patients, which allows us to protect the confidentiality of any single individual and to include several relevant examples in a more efficient manner.

C: (pulling her chair up to the table and demonstrating) Well, I usually sit like this, with my head resting on my right hand.

T: I notice that when you sit like that, the fingers of your hand are touching the hair on your temple.

C: Yeah, thats how the whole thing starts.

T: I think I can see where this is heading! Now, take me through this part really slowly, okay? I want this to be kind of like were going through a movie frame by frame, and youre telling me what happens in each of the frames. So here you are, at your desk studying after dinner, with the door closed. Your brothers are outside making noise. Youre resting your hand on your head. Whats going through your mind?

C: That I cant get any work done with them making all that noise!

T: You bet. What else?

C: Umm . . . that Im not going to get a good grade on my test and itll be their fault.

T: Okay. And what kinds of feelings are you having?

C: I guess Im feeling frustrated. And mad.

T: Frustrated and mad. I can see why, with all that noise out there. When you are feeling frustrated and mad, what does it feel like in your body?

C: I feel like Im clenching my teeth really hard, like my jaw hurts. And I get kind of a butterfly feeling in my stomach.

T: Anything else? Anything in the rest of your body?

C: Yeah, kind of a tense feeling in my shoulders and neck.

T: I wonder if you get kind of a wound-up feeling, like you cant relax?

C: Definitely. I feel like I want to jump up and down and scream!

T: As this is going on, are you having any urges to pull?

C: Maybe a little, but the urges get worse later.

T: Can you tell me what that urge is like?

C: Hmm . . . Its hard to describe. Its almost like a tingly feeling on my scalp, and Im paying a lot of attention to it, and Im starting to think about my head, and theres kind of a little voice inside my head thats telling me maybe Id feel better if I just pulled one hair.

Because Claudia reported that she pulls in multiple contexts, the therapist would go through these same kinds of questions for the other locations as well. Contrast Claudias early antecedents with those of Howard, described below.

Therapist (T): Id like to get a better understanding of how your hair pulling goes. Lets start by talking about the place where it occurs. Where is the location in which you are most likely to pull?

Howard (H): Thats easy. Really the only place I pull is when Im watching TV in the living room.

T: I see. Who is usually there with you?

H: Im always alone—Id be embarrassed to death if anyone saw me!

T: So where is everyone else at the time?

H: Well, my wife is usually in the kitchen making dinner, or maybe shes doing her sewing in this little room that she has up in the attic. My kids are usually outside playing in the yard.

T: Okay. When youre watching TV, where do you usually sit?

H: In my recliner. Its better for my back than the couch.

T: In the recliner, do you lean back and put the legs up?

H: I usually put the legs up, but I leave the back upright.

T: And where do you usually keep your hands?

H: Usually just like this (demonstrates), in my lap or maybe on the arms of the chair.

T: Okay. So Im starting to get a picture of how this goes. Youre sitting in the recliner with the legs up, watching TV, and your hands are resting on the arms of the chair or theyre in your lap. Youre by yourself. What are you thinking at the time?

H: Umm . . . I guess not much, really. Im just kind of watching the TV and not really thinking about anything.

T: Really focusing on the show?

H: Well, not really, more like Im just kind of zoned out and not really thinking about the show or about anything.

T: I think I get it. How do you feel at that time?

C: I guess Im feeling kind of bored, maybe kind of sleepy. The recliner is my favorite place to take a nap, you know, especially on Sunday when theres a football game on.

T: Me too! So kind of bored and sleepy, not really thinking about much of anything, kind of like you could fall asleep, do I have that right?

H: Yeah, thats about it.

T: Any physical sensations in your body that you notice? Like anything in your muscles, or in your chest, or stomach, or on your skin?

H: No, just kind of sleepy and bored.

T: Do you feel like you want to pull when youre sitting there?

H: No way! Im not even thinking about pulling, and if I did, pulling would be the last thing Id want to do.

As is clear from these descriptions, Claudia and Howard have different experiences that lead up to pulling. There are some similarities; for example, they both tend to engage in the problem behavior when alone, rather than in the presence of others, and they both choose body postures that may make it easier to start pulling. But Claudia tends to pull when she is angry and frustrated—that is, she is hyperaroused. And Claudia is also describing a clear pattern of thoughts and feelings about pulling, suggesting that her pulling may be *focused*. Howard, on the other hand, pulls when he is sleepy and bored, suggesting that *hypo*arousal may play a role. Howard is also unaware of pulling-related thoughts and feelings, suggesting *unfocused* pulling. We will learn more about these patterns below, as we come closer to the problem behavior itself.

Pre-Pulling Events. Having developed an understanding of the early antecedents, we now move on to discuss the events that immediately precede the problem behavior. These can include:

a. Preparatory "grooming"-like behaviors (e.g., touching hair or face)
b. Tactile or visual cues
c. Change in thoughts, feelings, or physiological sensations
d. Urges to pull

Below is a transcript of the assessment of Claudias pre-pulling events:

T: Okay, Claudia, youve described the setting very well, sitting there at the desk studying, with your hand in your head, feeling mad and tense, and maybe feeling a little bit of an urge to pull. Now I want us to let that movie go forward a bit to just before you actually pull. Whats happening now?

C: Well, I start running my fingers through my hair like this (demonstrates).

T: Kind of like youre combing your hair. What does that feel like to you?

C: The hair feels kind of nice going between my fingers, kind of relaxing.

T: What do you find relaxing about that? Is it something in the way your head feels, or something in the way your hair feels on your fingers?

C: Mostly the way my head feels right then; its like getting a scalp massage. But then I find a hair that doesnt feel right to me.

T: Doesnt feel right in what sense?

C: Could be anything, maybe its a little thicker than the rest, you know? Or maybe its curly where the rest of my hair is straight.

T: I see. And what do you do when you notice that one hair?

C: I rub it between my fingers (demonstrates rubbing thumb and forefinger together).

T: What does it feel like to rub the hair like that?

C: Its kind of a weird feeling on the tips of my fingers and then I really want to pull it.

T: You really want to pull it; how do you know when you want to pull it?

C: Well, its like I feel this pressure inside me, like in the middle of my chest, and the spot on my head where that hair is almost feels tingly, and I just feel like Im gonna explode if I dont pull that hair out.

Recall that Howards early antecedents were somewhat different from Claudias. Below, he describes that his pre-pulling events are also different.

T: Okay, so there you are, in the recliner with the legs up, watching TV, and feeling kind of bored and sleepy. No ones around. Lets discuss what happens right before you pull.

H: Thats tough to answer. I dont really know what happens before I pull. I seem to kind of lose track of things. I just look down and see that Ive been doing it again.

T: Are you aware of any new feelings, thoughts, sensations, or movements that might signal that youre about to begin pulling?

H: Well, I sort of notice that I start touching the hairs around my right knee, where I usually pull. But Im not really pulling them or even wanting to pull them. Im just kind of half noticing that there are some short, ingrown hairs there.

T: What does that feel like, to touch those short, ingrown hairs?

H: I dont like it. They feel rough and uneven to the touch.

Consistent with our analysis of early triggers, Claudia and Howard are describing a different functional sequence of behaviors, thoughts, emotions, and sensations. Both of them are engaging in what might be considered grooming-related behaviors (running fingers through the hair, or touching short, ingrown leg hairs), but they differ in terms of their internal experience of the event. Claudia is very focused on the behavior, is aware of her thoughts and feelings, and experiences an increased urge to pull following the tactile sensation of an irregular hair. Howard also seems somewhat drawn to the irregularity of his leg hairs, but less so, and he is still not experiencing urges. He remains relatively unfocused on his behavior.

Pulling Behaviors and Post-Pulling Events. The next area of assessment is the problem behavior itself and the events that follow it. As is the case with pre-pulling events, there is a substantial degree of heterogeneity in this area. A complete assessment of these events may include:

a. A detailed description of the behavior
b. Any change in thoughts, feelings, or physiological sensations during and immediately following the behavior
c. Visual behaviors: Does the patient look at the pulled hair? If so, at what aspect of the hair are they looking?
d. Tactile behaviors: Does the patient touch the pulled hair afterward? If so, how? What about this is potentially reinforcing?

e. Oral behaviors: Any behaviors that involve touching the pulled hair to the mouth, or biting or eating the hair.
f. How is the pulled hair discarded?
g. Any change in thoughts, feelings, or physiological sensations during and immediately following the post-pulling behaviors

Claudias report of her hair pulling and the events that follow are below:

T: Lets talk now about the pulling itself. Once youve isolated that irregular hair, what do you do?

C: Well, I just pull it out of my head.

T: Just one hair at a time, or do you pull out more than one at a time?

C: Just one at a time.

T: And do you pull it out quickly or slowly?

C: Kind of slowly. I dont really yank on it . . .I kind of like the way it feels when it comes out slowly.

T: What does that feel like to you?

C: I guess its kind of like theres a pulling sensation on my scalp that might last for half a second or so and then theres this release when the hair comes out.

T: A release—tell me about that part of it.

C: Its almost like I can feel a relaxing feeling on my scalp, I guess kind of like its soothing. And then it kind of feels like my whole body relaxes a little bit.

T: Does it hurt when you pull the hair?

C: Not really. It used to, a few years ago when I started. But it really doesnt now.

T: And how about those angry and frustrated feelings you had?

C: Its like I just forget about them and just feel that good relaxing feeling instead.

T: I see. So youve pulled a hair out; what do you do with the hair?

C: I kind of hang on to it for a while, sort of playing with it. I kind of wrap it around my fingers and maybe feel the end of it. And then I want to look at the hair too.

T: What are you looking for when you look at the hair?

C: I want to see if it still has the root on it.

T: What is it about the root?

C: Well, I want to see if it has a big white root on the end of it or not.

T: And if it does have that root on it?

C: Then its like I got a good one. Otherwise, I need to get another one and try again.

T: Sometimes kids with trich will put the hair up to their mouth. Ever do that?

C: (pause) Yeah. I didnt know other kids did that. That part of it is embarrassing.

T: I know you feel embarrassed, especially since you didnt know how common that is. But you know, a lot of kids will rub the hair on their lips, or theyll put the hair in their mouth, or bite the root off, or swallow the whole hair. Do you ever do those things?

C: Yeah, I rub the root part of the hair on my lower lip and then I bite the root off.

T: I see. Whats that like?

C: I guess it feels good on my lips, kind of like a little tickle. Its relaxing. And when I bite the root off, its kind of like Ive gotten that good one and now Im finishing the job, you know?

T: Sure. Do you swallow the root then?

C: Yeah.

T: And what happens to the rest of the hair?

C: I just drop it onto the floor next to me.

T: Do you stop then?

C: If I got a good one, maybe Ill stop for a minute or two. But then those feelings start to come back, those feelings like Im just tense and frustrated and want to pull another hair.

Howards description is different from Claudias:

T: Okay, you were telling me that you are aware of touching the short, ingrown hairs around your knee, and you were feeling how rough and uneven they were. What happens then?

H: I really dont know. Im just watching the TV and then I look down and I see that Ive done it.

T: What do you see?

H: Well, Ill notice that theres a little bald patch near my knee, and maybe Ill see some loose hairs on the chair next to me. Sometimes there will be a bloody spot on my knee, if some skin came off.

T: Whats that like, to see that?

H: Its like, "Oh damn, I did it again."

T: Does it hurt when you pull like that?

H: No, I dont even feel it, to be honest. I could pull a whole bunch of hairs, like 9 or 10, and not even be aware of it until I look down and see what Ive done.

T: I wonder whether sometimes it might feel good to you?

H: Not good, exactly . . . but I think that it feels a little better to get rid of the ingrown hairs. Its like my skin is a little smoother now, even though theres blood there, and even though I know those hairs will just grow back and bug me again. For the moment, its like I took off something that I didnt like having on me.

T: Is it that it looks better to you, or feels better?

H: A little of both. I like seeing my skin without those ingrown hairs; Id rather see blood on me than an ingrown hair. And it feels a little better too, like when I touch my knee, I dont feel those bumpy hairs. But of course, I know that makes no sense, because new hairs are just going to grow there.

T: What happens to those hairs you pulled out?

H: Well, sometimes when I realize that I pulled, Ill also notice that I still have a hair in my fingers.

T: I see. What do you do with it?

H: I kind of touch the end with the tip of my finger. The end is usually kind of sharp and stiff.

T: And whats it like to feel that end of the hair?

H: I guess it kind of feels interesting on my fingers.

T: And then what happens to the hair?

H: I just drop it onto the chair. It probably falls into the cushions or something. Id hate to see whats going on under those cushions (laughs)!

T: Ill bet (laughs)! Do you ever do anything else with it—for example, some people with a hair pulling problem will put the hair up to their mouth, maybe touch it to their lips. Ever do that?

H: Yuck! No, I just touch it and drop it.

Once again, we see that Claudia and Howard have a very different experience of pulling. Claudias pulling is very deliberate and focused, and she gets a clear feeling of relaxation from the sensation of pulling. Her pulling sequence is also notable for the presence of visual, tactile and oral behaviors that she finds rewarding. Howard, on the other hand, is largely unaware of the pulling itself, and denies experiencing any sensation of the pulling. However, he does find himself engaging in rewarding visual and tactile behaviors, and also reports some sense that it feels better to have the hairs removed.

FUNCTIONAL ANALYSIS OF HOWARD AND CLAUDIAS BEHAVIOR

Returning to the biopsychosocial model in Chapter 2, we can now fill in this model to arrive at a clearer understanding of Claudias and Howards pulling behavior. As we can see in Figures 4.1 and 4.2, although Claudia and Howard are both engaging in superficially similar behaviors (hair pulling), their behaviors occur in quite different functional contexts. By diagramming the behaviors along with their antecedents and

Figure 4.1 Functional diagram of Claudia's pulling behavior.

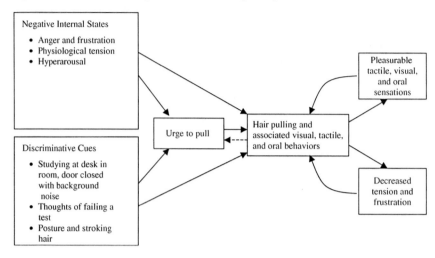

Figure 4.2 Functional diagram of Howard's pulling behavior.

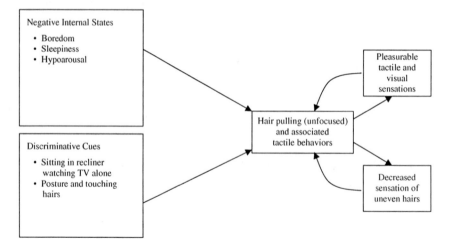

consequences, we gain a much richer understanding of how their pulling relates to internal and external triggers, as well as to alterations in internal sensations that might be reinforcing the problem. This functional understanding will come directly into play with the intervention strategies beginning in Chapter 7.

CHAPTER 5

WHAT SHOULD BE DONE?

Presentation of Treatment Alternatives

OVERVIEW

Our intent in this chapter is to present a summary of the TTM treatment outcome literature in adults as well as in children and adolescents in a clinically friendly manner. The information contained herein is especially relevant to present to patients early on in the process since they and their families will likely ask questions about the efficacy of the CBT approach being offered by clinicians using this manual, as well as the efficacy of other approaches such as pharmacotherapy and hypnotherapy. To facilitate communication of this information, a handout for patients and families is included in the appendix. As we will discuss, the treatment outcome literature on TTM remains underdeveloped, with only a few published RCTs with adults and none as yet in children and adolescents; this forces us to be more reliant on case studies and on clinical experience to guide treatment selection. Accordingly, we are cautious when we discuss our expectations for immediate and long-term efficacy of CBT as well as other approaches, and we emphasize that there are many unanswered questions about the relative efficacy of various CBT protocols versus other active treatments, the combined efficacy of CBT and pharmacotherapy, and the successful management of CBT partial response. What we do know from the work completed thus far is: 1) CBT appears to be a promising treatment; 2) evidence for the efficacy of pharmacotherapy is equivocal; and 3) relapse is a common problem in TTM, regardless of the treatment modality. Other treatments have also been brought to bear in TTM, yet the absence of scientifically acceptable studies of their efficacy limits what can be said about their potential benefits.

CBT PACKAGES

With respect to behavioral approaches and CBT packages, a variety of specific techniques have been applied, including awareness training, self-monitoring, aversion, covert sensitization, negative practice, relaxation training, habit reversal, competing response training, stimulus control, and overcorrection. Although the state of the CBT literature justifies only cautious recommendations, habit reversal incorporating competing response training, awareness training, and stimulus control are generally purported to be the core interventions for TTM, with other intervention strategies such as cognitive techniques to be used on an as-needed basis. As the review below emphasizes, however, more research is needed to dismantle the effectiveness of multi-component behavioral programs and inform the development of more efficacious and more durable cognitive-behavioral interventions. Based on our reading of the outcome literature, expert opinion in the field (e.g., Rothbaum & Ninan, 1999), and our own clinical experience with TTM, the CBT package we describe here focuses on the key elements of awareness training, stimulus control, competing response training, and maintenance/relapse prevention, with other techniques incorporated more on a case by case basis. We include the maintenance/relapse prevention strategies routinely in light of the long-term follow up data and based on our clinical experience with TTM patients suggesting that relapse is a common problem. Each of these core components and the modular components are described in detail in subsequent chapters and thus will not be elaborated upon here.

PHARMACOTHERAPIES

Five of the six pharmacotherapy RCTs conducted with TTM patients have examined the efficacy of serotonin reuptake inhibitors (SRIs). This trend reflects the view discussed above that TTM may be a variant of OCD, and thus should be responsive to the same medications that have proven efficacious with OCD (for reviews see Franklin, Riggs, & Pai, 2005; March, Franklin, Nelson, & Foa, 2001). More recently and, perhaps in response to the mixed results for the SRIs, other agents have been tried, such as opioid blockers (naltrexone), augmentation of SRI pharmacotherapy with atypical antipsychotics, and atypical antipsychotics alone. As yet there is no clear winner among these medications, and accordingly the field is now turning back to the experimental literature to inform pharmacotherapy treatment development (for a review see Franklin, Tolin, & Diefenbach, 2006). It is important to recognize, however, that many patients who present for CBT are already receiving pharmacotherapy, and the clinician should not assume that the medication is intended to reduce TTM symptoms per se. Instead, many of these patients are taking medication for comorbid conditions such as depression or anxiety disorders. Our research with OCD clinic outpatients suggests that patients who come in on medication and then receive CBT fare as well as those who receive CBT alone (Franklin, Abramowitz, Bux, Zoellner, & Feeny, 2002); those with repeated failed medication trials may have a less favorable prognosis but may still respond to CBT (Tolin, Maltby, Diefenbach, Hannan, & Worhunsky, 2004). We have insufficient clinical data to guide us regarding this issue in TTM. Nevertheless, when we encounter this situation in TTM patients we tend to be encouraging by saying we have little reason to believe that CBT and pharmacotherapy are incompatible.

SUMMARY OF TTM TREATMENT OUTCOME LITERATURE

Efficacy of Acute Treatment. Only seven randomized trials have been published to date, six of which included a control condition; none of these studies involved pediatric samples. There is an earlier and broader treatment literature generally made up of case studies, with progressively more controlled investigation in recent years (for a comprehensive review see Diefenbach et al., 2000). In general, knowledge about TTM treatments is limited by small sample sizes, lack of specificity regarding sample characteristics, non-random assignment to treatment, absence of long-term follow-up data, exclusive reliance on patient self-report measures, and lack of information regarding rates of treatment refusal and drop-out.

In the only published comparison of individual CBT to another psychosocial intervention, Azrin, Nunn, & Frantz (1980) found that habit reversal (HR) was more effective than negative practice: HR patients reported a 99% reduction in number of hair pulling episodes, compared to a 58% reduction for negative practice patients. Although encouraging, methodological issues limit the study's ultimate utility, including exclusive reliance upon patient self-report and the absence of a formal treatment manual to allow for replication. Group CBT was compared to supportive group therapy in an adult sample; results indicated that CBT was superior to the control condition at post-treatment, although some evidence of relapse in that group was evident (Diefenbach et al., 2006).

Of the six randomized controlled trials (RCTs) evaluating the efficacy of pharmacotherapy conducted to date, five involved serotonin reuptake inhibitors (SRIs): the selective serotonin reuptake inhibitors (SSRIs) or clomipramine, a tricyclic antidepressant with strong serotonergic properties. This reflects the

Table 5.1. Medications currently indicated for use with obsessive-compulsive disorder

Medication	Dose Range	Duration at Minimum Dose
Clomipramine (Anafranil ©)	150–250 mg	12 weeks
Fluoxetine (Prozac ©)	40–80 mg	12 weeks
Sertraline (Zoloft ©)	50–200 mg	12 weeks
Fluvoxamine (Luvox ©)	200–300 mg	12 weeks
Paroxetine (Paxil ©)	40–60 mg	12 weeks
Citalopram (Celexa ©)	40–60 mg	12 weeks

Adapted from Dougherty, D. D., Rauch, S. L., & Jenike, M. A. (2002). Pharmacological treatments for obsessive compulsive disorder. In P. E. Nathan & J. M. Gorman (Eds.), *A guide to treatments that work* (2nd ed., pp. 387–410). New York: Oxford University Press.

prevailing view that TTM is a variant of OCD and therefore ought to be responsive to the medications found helpful for that condition (for a review see March et al., 2001). Therapeutic dose ranges for TTM and other BFRBs have not been established. Table 5.1 shows medications that are indicated for use with OCD, and their therapeutic dose ranges for that disorder (Dougherty, Rauch, & Jenike, 2002).

In the first of these studies, Swedo et al. (1989) found clomipramine superior to desipramine at post-treatment in a double-blind crossover study involving fourteen adult women. In contrast, Christenson, Mackenzie, Mitchell, and Callies (1991) failed to demonstrate the superiority of fluoxetine over placebo in a double-blind crossover study. It is important to note that this finding did not occur because of a strong placebo response rate: neither fluoxetine nor placebo improved hair-pulling symptoms significantly. Streichenwein and Thornby (1995) extended the Christenson et al. (1991) study by lengthening the acute treatment phase and increasing the maximum fluoxetine dose to 80 mg, but they also failed to show any difference between fluoxetine and placebo in reducing hair pulling.

Two of the SRI RCTs included a direct comparison to cognitive-behavioral or behavioral protocols, information that is critical in informing patient choice between the two monotherapies. In the first of these, Ninan, Rothbaum, Marstellar, Knight, and Eccard (2000) found that, compared to clomipramine and placebo, CBT produced greater changes in hair pulling severity and associated impairment, and also yielded a significantly higher responder rate. Again in this study the medication monotherapy effects were not statistically significant, although there was a trend towards an advantage for clomipramine over placebo. Similarly, a recently published RCT found CBT superior to fluoxetine and waitlist, but failed to find a significant treatment effect for fluoxetine (van Minnen, Hoogduin, Keijsers, Hellenbrand, & Hendriks, 2003). Rothbaum et al. (1999) and van Minnen et al.'s (2003) findings suggest the superiority of CBT over SRI pharmacotherapy, although results from two studies do not a solid literature make, inviting neither grand sweeping statements nor especially confident conclusions. Taken together, results from the five controlled studies of SRIs are equivocal at best, and suggest that these medications are not especially potent in reducing TTM symptoms, at least in the short run.

In view of the small sample sizes and other methodological limitations of the pharmacotherapy studies conducted thus far, however, more controlled research should still be conducted to examine their efficacy more definitively. It may also be the case that the heterogeneity of TTM obscured treatment effects, and that subsets of TTM patients, more narrowly defined, might benefit from SRIs. Specifically, the studies discussed above did not limit sampling to those patients with strong negative affective triggers for pulling. Such patients might prove more responsive to these medications given their established efficacy in ameliorating symptoms of generalized anxiety disorder and depression (for reviews see Nemeroff & Schatzberg, 2002; Sussman & Stein, 2002). Thus, it might be informative to conduct SRI pharmacotherapy studies using samples of TTM patients with elevated anxiety and depression and an identified link between these negative affective states and their pulling.

As is clear from the above review, the TTM pharmacotherapy literature to date is both underdeveloped and equivocal. SRIs, the class of medication found routinely efficacious in OCD, have generally not proven efficacious for TTM. Perhaps, as we discussed in Chapter 2, important differences between OCD and TTM with respect to the role of negative and positive reinforcement in maintaining the two disorders, and the neurochemistry that underlies these processes, may account for this apparent discrepancy in treatment response. Intriguingly, naltrexone, an opioid blocking compound thought to decrease positive reinforcement by preventing the binding of endogenous opiates to relevant receptor sites in the brain, was found superior to placebo in reducing TTM symptoms (Christenson, Crow et al., 1994). In addition, several case studies have indicated that augmentation of SSRIs with atypical antipsychotics may be beneficial (e.g., Epperson, Fasula, Wasylink, Price, & McDougle, 1999), and a recent open trial suggested that olanzapine may be efficacious as a monotherapy for TTM (Stewart & Nejtek, 2003), although the absence of control conditions precludes clear interpretation of these studies. Clearly there is much more work to be done in the area of pharmacotherapy development and outcome evaluation, and the absence of a single RCT in pediatric TTM severely limits pharmacotherapy treatment recommendations that can be made to parents whose children suffer from this disorder.

Generally speaking, the limited and equivocal treatment literature strongly suggests that there is neither a universal nor complete response to *any* treatment for TTM. Given that monotherapy with CBT or pharmacotherapy is likely to produce only partial symptom reduction in the long run, these therapies might yield superior improvement when combined. Unfortunately, the absence of any controlled studies examining the efficacy of CBT, pharmacotherapy, and their combination weakens this claim considerably.

Long-term Outcome. Accumulating evidence from several open studies suggests that treatment response gained from pharmacotherapy may not be maintained in the long run. For example, an uncontrolled study by Pollard and colleagues (1991) indicated that the majority of a small sample of patients treated with clomipramine lost their treatment gains even while being maintained on a previously therapeutic dose. In addition, a retrospective study by Iancu, Weizman, Kindler, Sasson, and Zohar (1996) found that of patients receiving treatment with SRIs, 75% achieved a clinically significant response during the first two months, but symptoms returned to pretreatment levels during the third month despite continued medication. Following Swedo et al.'s (1989) positive study of clomipramine's acute efficacy, naturalistic follow-up suggested that long-term response varied widely and that overall a 40% reduction in symptoms was observed for those patients who participated in the four-year follow-up assessment (Swedo, Lenane, & Leonard, 1993).

Relapse also seems to be a concern following CBT discontinuation. Azrin, Nunn, & Frantz (1980) found that the effects of habit reversal training (HRT; see Chapter 9) were quite durable, in that the group who received HRT maintained their gains at 22-month follow-up, with patients reporting 87% reduction compared to pre-treatment. Although encouraging, methodological issues that affected the acute phase of the study, including exclusive reliance upon patient self-report also limit the utility of their findings at long-term follow-up, as did the substantial attrition (7 of 19) during the follow-up phase. An open study conducted by our research group examined immediate and long-term outcomes in patients who received nine weekly sessions of CBT (Lerner et al., 1998). Twelve of fourteen patients were classified as responders at post-treatment (50% or greater reduction on the NIMH-TSS), yet only 4 of 13 met this criterion an average of 3.9 years post-treatment. Keuthen, Fraim et al.'s (2001) naturalistic follow-up of patients who received state-of-the-art pharmacotherapy or behavior therapy further underscored concern about maintenance of gains following either form of treatment. Mouton and Stanley (1996) found that four of five patients benefited initially from group CBT, but only two of five patients maintained clinically significant gains at 6-month follow-up. Diefenbach et al. (2006) found that 22% of the patients receiving group CBT met criteria for clinically significant change in symptoms at post-treatment. However, at 1-month follow-up this percentage had declined to 12.5%, and by 3 and 6- month follow-up, none of the patients scored in the range for clinically significant change. In our open trial of CBT for children and adolescents with TTM (Tolin et al., 2006), of the 12 patients classified as "responders" at the end of active treatment (week 8), 3 (25.0%) lost that designation during the follow-up phase. Of the 17 patients classified as "responders" at the end of the relapse prevention phase (week 16), 4 (23.5%) lost this designation during follow-up.

OTHER TREATMENT APPROACHES

A wide variety of treatments have been applied to TTM, but in general the efficacy of treatments other than CBT and SRIs has not been tested using scientifically accepted methods and thus strong conclusions about their benefit cannot be drawn. Nevertheless, we have seen several patients who described positive responses to hypnotherapy, several others who reported that psychodynamic approaches were helpful for them, and have met many others still who swear by other alternative interventions (for a review of alternative therapies posed for TTM see Penzel, 2003). Convergent with the outcome literature, we have had our fair share of patients who either did not respond to either CBT or SRI, or who relapsed after treatment discontinuation. Open-mindedness to new possibilities is not incompatible with scientific rigor, and it is clear that the collective response to CBT and SRIs documented thus far is far from universal or complete. Clinically, we recommend a supportive stance whenever our patients, prospective patients, or their families describe a new treatment method they have encountered and are considering. We view their search for the "magic bullet" as a reflection of the struggle they are enduring with TTM or, perhaps even more sadly, watching a loved one endure. Thus, we encourage open discussion with patients about the treatment alternatives they encounter. That said, we owe our patients and their families the best advice we can provide, which includes educating them about the scientific status of various interventions (cf. Lilienfeld, Lynn, & Lohr, 2003). We do not hesitate, therefore, to inform patients that treatments that sound too good to be true usually are. As space engineer James Oberg reminded us, "Keeping an open mind is a virtue, but not so open that your brains fall out."

It is also important to consider that the efficacy of *any* treatment for TTM cannot be measured simply by reductions in hair pulling: the negative social and emotional consequences of TTM may also be appropriately targeted in treatment, and some prospective patients who are simply not ready to work directly on the hair pulling may benefit from treatment of these other difficulties. One of our adolescent patients who did not make substantial amount of progress in reducing her hair pulling reported that she viewed the treatment as helpful nevertheless, since she now better understood the disorder, no longer blamed herself for being "weird" or "weak," knew that she was not the only person who engaged in this habit, felt supported by the therapist, and learned about the various procedures that she could implement when she decided the time was right. Such contributions by the therapist should not be underestimated, as the therapist has much more to offer than mere technique (Tolin & Hannan, 2005). We try to convey when we meet new prospective patients that CBT requires a substantial amount of effort and that the costs of these efforts should be considered as treatment alternatives are weighed.

CONVEYING INFORMATION ABOUT TREATMENT ALTERNATIVES TO PATIENTS AND FAMILIES

Susan is a 37-year-old married woman with two children. From her initial evaluation session, we determined that Susan's pulling began during elementary school and was confined to eyebrows and eyelashes at that time but since late adolescence has also included scalp hair. Her pulling was primarily unfocused at first, and occurred mostly when she was alone in her office at work (she worked as a supervisor in the Human Resources department of a large company) or when she was reading or watching television prior to going to bed. She tended to roll the pulled hair in her fingers briefly and then discard it, and she had noticed that her pulling tended to increase when she was facing deadlines at work or when life at home was more stressful. Susan was considering a course of CBT monotherapy, and was interested in hearing more about how the CBT program worked.

S: So it sound like you think that I have trich, and that there are a few options for me to think about.

T: Yeah, I think it's pretty clear that this is trich, and from what I gather it's the main problem going on for you right now, other than your sense of being stretched too thin by the demands of day-to-day life.

S: That sounds just about right. I've noticed too that the pulling has been worse since my youngest started school this fall.

T: It's one more thing that you have to attend to, and you've got a lot going on already from what you've said. The workload's been heavier too since September, right?

S: It has, and the time I spend pulling at work stresses me out even more.

T: Which probably increases the urges to pull, too.

S: Yup.

T: Well, as we've discussed we have a CBT program here that focuses on teaching you to become more aware of the particulars of your pulling pattern, and then to use specific behavioral methods to make your environment less conducive to pulling and to give you alternative things to do that are both satisfying and incompatible with pulling. There's other stuff we sometimes include too, like stress management techniques for people whose pulling seems to be related to their feeling frazzled.

S: I suppose I might be a candidate for that? (laughs)

T: You certainly have some of the risk factors for that, and I think we'd learn a lot about the particulars through the awareness training part of the program. The program is laid out to include weekly treatment for about eight weeks, and then we'll see where we are.

S: You think I'll be done in eight weeks?

T: I think it depends on what you mean by "done." I tend to think about TTM as something that people have to work on over the course of a lifetime, so I don't think it's realistic to think that we can eradicate it completely in eight weeks. However, the core elements of the CBT program can be taught in that amount of time, and also ought to allow you a good opportunity to practice the techniques while we're working together weekly. After that, we usually spread sessions out to every other week to give you more time to put it all into practice and to really get into the habit of using the strategies you've learned. Like this program, the CBT programs that have been tested in treatment outcome studies are short-term therapies. The idea is that what you learn in CBT will help reduce the symptoms in the short run and, maybe more importantly, put you in a better position to gain better control over trich in the long run. We have had some people make really great progress in eight weeks and maintain their gains, but what we know from research studies and from our clinical experience is that most folks who have trich probably don't ever lose the urge completely, even if they get treated. The studies of CBT that have been done so far do tell us that people on average make pretty good gains, though, and that CBT works better than control treatments and seems to be better than the antidepressant medications alone.

S: So, if I were able to stop pulling hair from this treatment, how long would that last?

T: So far, the best evidence we have suggests that, regardless of what kind of treatment is used, people who respond well to treatment are still at risk of having their hair pulling start to come back later on. It doesn't happen to everyone, but it happens enough that we should anticipate it and prepare for it. You and I might find it helpful to plan on having some additional sessions in the future if you notice the problem starting to get worse.

S: What happens in the treatment sessions?

T: In some ways this treatment is like a lot of psychotherapies, in that you'll let me know what's been going on with you during the week and we'll discuss how you're feeling about things. In other ways it's a little bit like going to see a coach or a piano teacher, in that I'll try to teach you what we know about trich and its treatment and you'll get the chance to put the lessons into practice from week to week. Then when we meet again each week we'll see how the techniques are working, and troubleshoot when we see things that need to be addressed. It's similar to learning a new skill with a coach or a piano teacher in that most of the real work takes place not during the instruction session itself, but when you're practicing the things we're working on between the sessions.

S: I've also heard about the medicines that affect serotonin – do you think I should be on one of those while I'm doing CBT?

T: These medicines haven't proven especially helpful in reducing trich symptoms, although they're often used when people have other symptoms as well as the TTM, such as anxiety or depression. Also, even though there are some reasons to think that combined treatment might be best, believe it or not, that hasn't been studied thoroughly yet. In anxiety disorders, which are at least somewhat similar to trich, combined treatments generally haven't been found to be much better than CBT alone, so we generally don't say that people have to do both.

S: I've also seen on some website that there's some kind of diet that's supposed to be very helpful for trich – do you know about that?

T: There are a lot of different things that people try when they're attempting to work on reducing their trich symptoms, including diets, diet supplements, herbal remedies and a variety of other things. I'd also say there are probably lots of treatments out there that might work that we don't know about yet. What I'd say about them in general is that they haven't been carefully studied as yet, meaning using randomization to control groups like pill placebos or, in the case of a diet, a comparison group of people with trich that didn't get the diet. It doesn't mean that any individual won't do better after they try one of these treatments, only that we don't have strong evidence in support of them as yet. It's also the case that if we don't have good studies we won't know why something works, which is another problem. The treatment studies tell us about the probable outcomes with a particular treatment, and the information we have so far indicates that CBT is probably going to be helpful, whereas we have much less information to go on with the untested therapies. I'd also say that if someone says that a single treatment is going to completely eliminate trich forever they're probably overstating things: trich is a complex and chronic problem, and unlikely therefore to be easily and completely eliminated.

WHAT DO WE NEED TO KNOW?

Frequently and Infrequently Asked Questions

Successful treatment is predicated on a collaborative working relationship with the patient. Thus, it is critical that the patient be well informed about his/her illness and its treatment. We find it helpful to allow ample time prior to the beginning of treatment to solicit questions from the patient. When addressed before treatment, they set the stage for a positive collaboration. When a patient's questions are not raised or answered prior to treatment, they are likely to come up during the treatment itself, which can often distract from the main goals of the intervention. Some patients may never ask the questions that are on their minds; we suspect that these patients are at higher risk for nonadherence or dropout. Therefore, we often begin this conversation by reminding the patient that there are no "dumb" questions and that many people have questions that they might not feel completely comfortable asking, only to find out that their concerns are actually quite common. Some of the frequently- and infrequently-asked questions we have encountered, and our usual responses, are listed below.

Q: Why do I pull my hair?

A: That's a tough question to answer. We don't know all of the reasons why you pull, but we have some good ideas about some of the reasons. The part we find hardest to answer is why you started pulling in the first place. It's quite possible that there is a genetic component to this, and that some people are naturally predisposed to pulling. However, genetics alone don't fully explain it. You didn't inherit this problem in the same way that you inherited, say, your eye color. More likely, you inherited some characteristics of how your brain works that made it easier for you to develop this problem under certain circumstances. Those circumstances might include stressful life events such as [give examples from patient's history]. So most likely, this problem comes from a combination of genetic and environmental factors. What we know a bit more about, however, is how this problem is maintained. The things that started this problem are not necessarily the same things that keep it going. As you can see in this diagram (showing the diagram in Figure 1), over time your brain has learned to associate certain situations, activities, thoughts, or feelings, with pulling. So whenever you're in that situation, or feeling that feeling, your brain tells you it's time to pull. Sometimes you'll experience that association in the form of an urge; sometimes you won't feel the urge but your brain will just get your fingers to start doing it. When you pull, it changes the way you feel. Maybe it makes some bad feelings go away for a little bit, or maybe it gives you a pleasant feeling. Either way, these feelings reward the action because your brain learns that it can make itself feel better by making you pull. Of course, these feelings don't last very long, so after a while you don't feel quite as good and you feel that need to pull again. So we think that the problem is maintained because your brain has learned two things: first, that when you're in [name a situation from the patient's experience], it's time to pull; and second, when you pull, you can feel a little bit better.

Q: Will this problem ever get better? Can it be cured?

A: We find that most people with this problem who get the right kind of treatment see a noticeable decrease in their pulling, so you have a very good chance of seeing this problem get better. Of course, no treatment will work for everyone, and so you and I need to keep an eye on how you are responding to this treatment. If it doesn't seem to be working, we'll discuss whether it's time to change strategies until we find something that does work for you. It's important to be realistic in our expectations, though, because no "cure" for this has been developed yet. Most people that we see don't stop pulling completely; rather, their pulling decreases to a level that they find manageable. You should also know that once someone is finished with treatment, even when the treatment went really well, they are always going to be at increased risk for pulling again. So it would be unrealistic for us to expect that you'll stop pulling 100% and never start again, although that would be great if it happened. What's important is that when you do find yourself pulling, that you put it in the proper perspective. Your initial thought might be, "Oh, no, I'm doing it again! My treatment didn't work and the situation is hopeless!" But you can respond to that thought by telling yourself, "Hey, this is just a lapse. I knew this was likely to happen. I'm not thrilled about this, but it's not the end of the world and it doesn't mean the situation is hopeless. It just means that I need to be more vigilant in applying the strategies I learned in my treatment, and maybe call my therapist if I can't handle it on my own."

Q: Am I the only one who does this?

A: I hear that one all the time! You are definitely not the only one who does this. We don't have precise epidemiological data, but some studies suggest that up to 10% of people pull their hair at least some time, and about 1% have some hair loss because of pulling. That means that one out of every ten people pulls their hair, and one out of every hundred pulls hair to the point of hair loss. That's a lot of people! People with this problem often want to keep it a secret, though, so they don't tell anyone about it. You might even know some people who do this, even if they haven't told you. They might hide their bald patches under a wig, or only pick skin that is covered by clothes.

Q: Is this a chemical imbalance?

A: Well, yes and no. Certainly your brain chemistry is involved in pulling. When you feel an urge to pull, or when you get that pleasurable sensation after pulling, what you're really feeling is the chemistry of your brain influencing other parts of your body. On the other hand, though, everything we think, feel, and do is the result of a "chemical imbalance!" If you take piano lessons, for example, those lessons actually change the chemistry of your brain a little bit, because it's those chemicals that will cause you to remember how to hold your fingers on the keys, how to play chords, and so on. But it would be kind of strange to say that knowing how to play the piano is the result of a chemical imbalance, even though that would be technically true. There are just better ways of explaining it. We'd probably find it more sensible to say that the person knows how to play piano because they learned how to play piano. In your case, it might be accurate to say that a chemical imbalance plays a role in the beginning and the maintenance of your problem. But it would also be accurate, and perhaps more informative in some cases, to say you learned to pull. Neither one is more true than the other; they're both true. It's just a difference in the level of analysis we want to use.

Q: Do I have a problem of willpower?

A: Willpower is not a particularly useful way of explaining this problem. None of us are 100% in control of our actions, 100% of the time. Even our "freedom of choice" is influenced by factors outside ourselves. When I got up this morning, I had cereal for breakfast. There was a box of corn flakes and a box of oatmeal on the shelf, and I chose the corn flakes. Sounds like I made my own decision, didn't it? But my choice was partly determined by what was on the shelf. I wasn't able to choose, for example, raisin bran, because that wasn't available to me. I had a cup of coffee, too. Did I make my own decision? Partly, because I knew I wanted a cup of coffee. But I also knew that I drink coffee every morning, and I'm in the habit of doing that, plus I knew that if I didn't have that coffee I'd be tired and cranky today. So even though I was in charge of my decisions, my actions were influenced by other things. That's what's going on with you. You are in charge of your behaviors, and yet you are not in control of them. Your actions are being influenced by your habits, your learning, and the way you feel when you try not to do them. So in this treatment, we're not looking to build willpower. The fact that you've come here tells me you have plenty of that. Instead, we're going to try to increase your sense of control over your behavior, so that we limit the degree to which these other factors influence you.

Q: Is hair pulling a sign of serious mental illness? Am I crazy?

A: Definitely not. Most of the people I've met with this problem are perfectly normal people. They just have a problem that they have a hard time getting control of. A lot of the time, people with pulling problems will also have problems of depression or anxiety, but that's a far cry from being "crazy." Most of the time, when people use a word like "crazy," they are referring to a very serious mental illness called schizophrenia. People with schizophrenia usually have very dramatic and noticeable symptoms, such as hearing voices, or believing that someone is monitoring them through their television. In other words, it's pretty hard to miss, and you would most certainly know if you had those symptoms. Sometimes people worry that someday their pulling will turn into that kind of problem. But there's no evidence at all that this occurs.

Q: Does hair pulling mean that something terrible happened to me in my past that I can't remember?

A: It's often tempting to guess that your pulling is a sign of terrible trauma in your past. But the evidence doesn't seem to support that kind of association. Most people who pull didn't have a horrible trauma, and most people who have a horrible trauma don't pull. Furthermore, although it might be possible for someone to have a horrible experience that they can't remember, in most cases, when someone experiences a traumatic event, they remember it quite clearly. So there's no reason to believe that your pulling is a sign of some hidden past trauma.

Q: Will my hair grow back? Have I done permanent damage?

A: Hair usually grows back if you can leave it alone. It often takes a while for it to grown in, and when it grows it's often uneven, patchy, or itchy. Unfortunately, these are exactly the kind of things that trigger a lot of people to pull in the first place, so many people pull out the hair that's trying to grow back in. If you can refrain from pulling, chances are your hair will grow in. The bottom line is that you will never know how your hair will look until you let it heal itself.

Q: Is this an addiction?

A: In some ways, pulling is like an addiction. We might find it helpful to think of this as a case of you getting "hooked" on pulling, and the way it makes you feel.

Just like a person with an addiction, you find it difficult to do just a little of this, because the good feeling doesn't last, so you have to do more and more. But we should be careful to keep in mind that calling it an addiction doesn't mean that you can't learn to regain control over the behavior.

Q: Do I have OCD?

A: There's a lot of disagreement about that. Some psychologists and psychiatrists think that trichotillomania is part of what is called an "OCD spectrum," meaning it's related to OCD. There certainly are some similarities between this problem and OCD. Both problems are characterized by a repetitive behavior that you can't fully control. There may be some genetic similarities, too; people with pulling are often related to people with OCD. From a medication standpoint, the medications that are helpful for OCD might be helpful for pulling, which might mean that similar brain activity is involved. But there are some important differences, too. In my thinking, the most important difference is that people with OCD do their behaviors for a very different reason than you do. A person with OCD who washes his hands all the time, for example, is doing so because he is fearful that if he stops, he'll contract a disease and die. A person with OCD who checks the stove over and over again is afraid that if she doesn't do it perfectly, her house will burn down. So most people with OCD are doing their compulsions because they are afraid, and their compulsion helps them feel a little less afraid. People who pull, on the other hand, aren't doing it because they are afraid. Most of the time, they find that pulling makes them feel good, or maybe makes them feel less bored, or sad, or stressed out. So rather than thinking of this problem as OCD, I think we'll find it more useful to think of it as a habit that has gotten out of your control and has become a burden for you.

PART 2

TREATMENT: CORE ELEMENTS

CHAPTER 7

YOU CAN'T FIGHT WHAT YOU CAN'T SEE:

Awareness Training and Self-Monitoring

INTRODUCTION TO AWARENESS TRAINING AND SELF-MONITORING

We discussed in the assessment section of this book the importance of assisting the patient in becoming more aware of the very first signs of the behavioral chain of pulling. TTM in many cases is characterized by "unfocused" pulling, which further underscores the importance of this task. Because stimulus control and competing response procedures can be put in place in "high risk" situations only once those situations have been identified, instruction in awareness training begins in the first clinical session after the assessment has been completed and the patient has agreed to initiate CBT. Self-monitoring is one of the core techniques used to improve awareness, although we also discuss below other methods that serve this same function and thus fall under the umbrella of awareness training. Perhaps because it increases attention to the problem behaviors themselves, the context in which they occur, and the consequences they elicit, self-monitoring has been found to be an effective intervention in and of itself for appetitive behaviors such as overeating (e.g., Romanczyk, 1974) and smoking (e.g., Abrams & Wilson, 1979). We make clear up front that self-monitoring data will be reviewed with the therapist in each session, and this contingency may increase the patient's motivation to pay attention to the details of their pulling (Tolin & Hannan, 2005). Moreover, the monitoring data are also a potential source of positive reinforcement when plotted on graphs for the patient to view their progress. With our younger patients we often make graphs of self-monitoring data in colorful and attractive styles likely to be perceived as pleasant, and encourage the patient's active participation in the creation and decoration of these charts.

ORIENTING PATIENTS TO SELF-MONITORING

The rationale we provide for self-monitoring usually begins with an analogy about carefully examining a phenomenon to what is happening first before deciding how to respond appropriately. Sports metaphors work especially well for this purpose (e.g., football coaches and players "watching film" to identify their next opponent's tendencies), but of course these metaphors should always be tailored to the interests and developmental level of the individual. It is also important to feed back to the patient the information that has been gleaned already from the assessment. With one of our patients, a 45-year woman old named Maureen, the summary of the assessment materials and initial description of self-monitoring went as follows:

T: From our first session last week we determined that your pulling tends to happen at night after you've put the kids to bed, it starts usually when you're in bed reading, there's usually a few minutes of touching your hair with your left hand first, and you experience that "keyed-up " feeling right before you begin pulling. Does that sound right to you?

M: Yes, plus sometimes when I'm driving and I'm stuck in traffic.

T: That's right. We've learned some important things already about your pulling pattern, but in order to put ourselves in the best position to really do something about it we'll have to get one or two steps ahead of it. One of the best ways to do that is to begin to keep track of trich as it's occurring, and that's why I want you to begin self-monitoring after our session today ends (takes out two self-monitoring sheets and hands one to Maureen). I've created this sheet for you on which you can record the situations in which you are pulling, any emotions, feelings, or thoughts you noticed right before a particular pulling episode started, whether or not you touched your head a few minutes before you pulled the first one, plus the number of hairs pulled per episode.

M: Looks like a lot to keep track of.

T: It is, but it gets a lot easier once you get used to using the forms, and the information we'll get from this will be really helpful in developing a comprehensive treatment plan.

M: Can I do this at the end of the day instead of throughout the day?

T: I'd suggest that you try as best you can to monitor right as it's happening, since you'll be more accurate that way. There's also a side benefit of doing this, which is that it may make you more aware of what you are doing; that might be helpful in your efforts to stop pulling. You wouldn't get that benefit, though, if you waited until the end of the day to complete the form.

M: What about when I'm in public or going from place to place? I don't want people to see what I'm doing since most of the people I'm around probably don't even know that I have this problem.

T: Good question. This comes up enough in our work with trich that we even have these handy folders in which you can put the sheet so that you can be discreet about the monitoring when that's needed (hands folder to Maureen). Just for practice, why don't we try to use this sheet to record whatever you remember about the last time you pulled – can you recall when that was?

M: It was last night, after my husband went to bed.

T: Well let's get that written down under the "Where" column. (hands pen to Maureen for her to record pulling episode.) Do you remember what time that was?

M: It was pretty late – I think Letterman was already on.

T: After the monologue?

M: No, probably during – I went to bed before he did the Top Ten List.

T: Good, that narrows the window down a bit. Do you remember if you were touching your hair before the pulling started?

M: Yeah, I was sitting on the couch and had my elbow on the armrest with my head leaning on my hand.

T: Feeling tired?

M: Yeah, I think so.

T: What were you thinking about prior to pulling?

M: Just thinking about whether my daughter had a clean shirt for school – not much else. Do people usually say that they're thinking about pulling before they start?

T: It varies some, but actually lots of people with trich don't report much thinking about pulling immediately preceding pulling – some say that they're wrapped up in other things like watching TV or talking on the phone, almost like it's happening outside of their awareness.

M: That sounds like what happens to me.

T: Do you recall any physical feelings or sense of tension during that time?

M: More like an itch, I think.

T: Do you remember how many hairs you pulled?

M: No idea – probably not too many since I was down there for only about ten minutes or so. I see here that you want me to write down the number of hairs that I pulled – I can see why this is hard to do long after the fact.

*T: Exactly – when are recording in real time we'll have that information right
here on the sheet for us to review, and we'll begin to see the kinds of patterns that
will help us anticipate when pulling is likely to be a problem, plus we'll learn
more about the context in which it occurs. All that information will be really helpful as we create our battle plan.*

SAVING PULLED HAIRS

At this time we also introduce another technique designed to improve awareness of
pulling and to serve as a check for the patient on the accuracy of self-monitoring,
which is the collection of pulled hairs in an envelope that will be brought to each
of the subsequent treatment sessions. Understandably this is a technique that
causes some discomfort for patients and occasionally for therapists, but we tend
to include it for several reasons. First, it provides another objective measure of
pulling that might improve the accuracy of self-monitoring data given that the
therapist will ask to inspect the sheets and the collected hairs. Second, getting up
and placing the pulled hairs immediately into an envelope will curtail some of
the post-pulling behaviors that some patients find very reinforcing, such as
rolling the hair between their fingers, rubbing it on their faces and lips, biting off
the root, sticking the root to a piece of paper, or ingesting the hair. Of course,
ingestion of hair precludes saving the hair for some patients, but these patients
should nevertheless be given the instructions to immediately place pulled hairs
into the envelope as a stimulus control method, since we wish to decrease positive reinforcement associated with the hair pulling process. It is important to
underscore that this technique is not designed to be embarrassing or humiliating
to patients, but rather to serve these other purposes. We explain how the hair will
be used in session as well: as we are reviewing the self-monitoring sheet the
envelope will be opened and visually inspected; once the monitoring sheets have
been discussed and the accuracy of the data contained therein is estimated, the
hairs are discarded in the therapist's wastebasket and the session continues. For
some patients this rationale and description is still insufficient in helping hem
overcome their sense of embarrassment about having to collect, examine, and
also bring in saved hairs to the treatment session. In such cases, we encourage
therapists to use their clinical judgment to determine if this aspect of awareness
training should be omitted. In our clinical experience this is a relatively rare
occurrence, and we tend to be somewhat matter of fact about the request so as to
avoid infusing the interaction with our own trepidation about this element of
treatment. It is not uncommon in our clinical experience for patients to tell us,
after treatment, that saving pulled hairs was one of the key ingredients that
helped them stop pulling.

SELF-MONITORING'S OTHER FUNCTIONS IN TTM

We emphasize here that self-monitoring improves awareness of the pulling habit and as such should be strongly emphasized. However, self-monitoring also serves other functions that we discuss with patients. For example, self-monitoring serves a stimulus control function in that patients who are following instructions to record pulling behavior as it occurs need to stop their pulling to go and get their folder and then write down the relevant data on the recording sheet. It can also be conceptualized as a form of competing response: the patient who leaves the high-risk situation to retrieve their folder now also has a pen in their hand as they are writing, which can then be used as an object to fiddle with in order to keep their hands busy. We explained these functions to an 11-year-old boy named Keith who happened to be a very enthusiastic sports fan:

T: So you see now why it's so important for you to try to record the pulling right as it's happening?

K: Yeah, 'cause it's hard to remember what happened an hour ago and you want it to be right.

T: Yeah, it's important that we get it down as accurately as possible, since the more we learn about your pulling pattern the better off we'll be in terms of figuring out what to do and when to do it with the other techniques you'll learn.

K: Yeah.

T: Also if you really think about it self-monitoring serves another purpose too, which is breaking up trich's rhythm. Remember how you said that sometimes you just get into a zone when you're pulling? One of the things that self-monitoring will do is give you a way to break that rhythm by getting up from where you're sitting, go and open you folder, and concentrate on what was just happening. You don't want trich to get a good rhythm going, since that's often the time when people tell me that they pull the most hair. Maybe you can try to think about it like the way hitters in baseball try to throw off a good pitcher's rhythm by stepping out of the batter's box.

K: Yeah, they ask the umpire for time, step out, rub dirt on their hands, adjust their batting gloves, all sorts of stuff.

T: Right, and a lot of that is done to throw off the pitcher, get them out of their rhythm. There was a guy who used to play for Texas when I was a kid named Mike Hargrove who used to drive pitchers crazy doing that – he earned the nickname "The Human Rain Delay" for all of his antics, and sometimes pitchers would make mistakes to him because they just wanted to get him out of there. Maybe we can get you to be "The Human Rain Delay" when it comes to trich – break trich's rhythm, and make sure you don't go right back to the place you were pulling after you monitor.

K: I should probably keep my folder across the room from my bed so it forces me to get up.

T: Exactly. Now you also told me that you pull when you're watching TV, right?

K: Yes, sometimes.

T: If we want the self-monitoring to also work to break trich's rhythm there, where should you put the folder?

K: Maybe leave it in my room and get it when I notice that I'm pulling?

T: That depends – is your room right next to the family room where the big TV is?

K: No it's upstairs.

T: Which means you might not want to go and make all that effort to go get it? I know if I was watching the Red Sox I might be tempted to wait until between innings to make the trip upstairs.

K: Then how about on top of the TV?

T: That would be better, I think – it will serve the same purpose but will be more likely to be something you'd do right away.

K: Yeah, I think so.

T: Good, why don't we try that this week, and we'll see how it works.

K: OK.

MAKING USE OF SELF-MONITORING DATA

Having given clear instructions about the rationale for and importance of self-monitoring and collection of saved hairs, the therapist's crucial next task is to make effective use of the data. Optimally the patient will return with sheets on which data were collected in real time, hairs collected in the envelope that had been provided for this purpose, and filled with new insights about the nature of their pulling; indeed, we have had many cases in which the early awareness training set the stage for successful implementation of stimulus control and competing response training, which are both facilitated by knowledge of the high risk times for pulling. In this situation the therapist should enter the data on number of hairs pulled in the past week into a computer database such as PowerPoint or Excel, or onto a graph drawn by hand (or if working with younger patients allow the child to do so if they are so inclined), and then inspect the sheet for the early signs of a pattern to pulling, such as by location (e.g., cubicle in school library), time of day, or consistent affective trigger (e.g., boredom). We emphasize that the pulling profile won't always emerge immediately, but that by collecting such accurate data the patient is putting him/herself in a great position to detect patterns and then respond based on what the data tell us. We are effusive with our praise when patients do a good job with monitoring early on in treatment, since we recognize that the monitoring is the foundation upon which the rest of the treatment must rest. With younger children we are quick to supply external reinforcers for accuracy, such as colorful stickers with which to decorate their folders and monitoring sheets. Occasionally patients will be disappointed that they have continued to pull despite the fact that treatment has already begun, and we let them know that this is to be expected. On rare occasions we have encountered patients whose pulling virtually ceases after the monitoring procedures are put in place, since they are reluctant to write down the details of pulling episodes or to collect saved hairs. More often than not these patients are still experiencing urges to pull, and thus treatment should proceed according to plan despite this dramatic reduction in pulling. In our experience this kind of reactivity to the monitoring task does not usually last for more than a few weeks, and thus is not a reason to pronounce a patient "cured" and discontinue the treatment prematurely. However, it is generally good clinical practice to delay new interventions until a stable baseline of the behavior has been established (i.e., it is clear that the behavior will not improve without the intervention; cf. Barlow & Hersen, 1984).

The clinician should carefully examine the data to determine whether the patient knows (or could be taught to know) in advance whether he/she might pull. Primarily unfocused pullers may be less likely to know at this stage of treatment, but inquire nevertheless. As emphasized above, these precursors can be physical feelings (e.g., itching at the pulling site), environmental (e.g., watching TV alone at night in room), behavioral (e.g., touching or stroking hair before pulling is initiated), or emotional (e.g., when tense/anxious about school). Continued self-monitoring will provide more information about this as the treatment unfolds, but it is useful to inquire in some detail in the first session. In addition, it is important to inquire about different environments (e.g., school vs. home) as well as different areas within environments (e.g., math class vs. gym class). These early discussions set the stage for the kind of "sleuthing" that we want our TTM patients to engage in – indeed, with our younger patients we make analogies to being detectives to determine when TTM strikes so that we can anticipate its next move and "catch it in the act."

We also make use of the collected hairs as part of the monitoring review, quickly examining to see if the number of pulled hairs recorded on the monitoring sheet over the past week corresponds roughly to the amount of hair in the envelope. If there is much more hair in the envelope than was recorded on the sheet the clinician should inquire about whether each pulling episode was tracked. Sometimes we find that the envelope was kept right next to the patient in an environment where they tend to pull often (e.g., couch) whereas the monitoring sheet remained in a less accessible place. In this situation we reinforce efforts to save hairs but emphasize that the envelope should be moved further away, giving the patient an incentive to break the rhythm of pulling by getting up, retrieving the envelope and the folder, and recording the pulling episode immediately. Alternatively, we have seen some patients whose recorded number of hairs greatly exceeds the amount in the envelope, which can sometimes signify reluctance to place hairs in the envelope, inadequate planning (e.g., envelope kept in car when pulling takes place in office), or possibly previously undisclosed trichophagia. It is important to inquire gently about all of these possibilities when there is a discrepancy, and to encourage collaborative problem solving when such difficulties are encountered.

BARRIERS TO SELF-MONITORING

The clinician's task is more complicated when the patient returns to the next session with partially complete or missing monitoring sheets. A problem solving approach is encouraged, as is a functional analysis: it is simply insufficient and unhelpful to deem this behavior as "non-compliance" and put the problem squarely in the lap of the patient. Instead, these difficulties should be conceptualized as a problem in the therapy that requires active participation of the therapist and patient working as a team towards a productive solution (for a detailed discussion of successfully negotiating motivational issues see Chapter 11). First, we elicit from the patient their account of why the monitoring task proved difficult, and we use that discussion to generate potential solutions. With Jennifer, a 12-year-old girl with eyebrow and eyelash pulling, the discussion went as follows:

T: I see that you've got your folder with you, and your envelope too – why don't we take a look at them and see what they can teach us about your trich.

J: (Clutching folder and looking at floor) I don't think they're going to teach us too much – I did some pulling this week, but I didn't always write it down. I also didn't put the hairs into the envelope.

T: Well, I've found here that it's often hard to get going with the monitoring stuff – why don't we try to think about what got in the way, and see if we can figure out ways to make it easier.

J: (Makes direct eye contact) OK.

T: Good – let's start with the folder, OK? Before we look at what you were able to record, can you make a guess about how accurate it is?

J: It was pretty good the first few days, but then the weekend came and after that I think I pulled a couple of times but didn't write it down.

T: First let's think about the days when you think the monitoring was pretty accurate – where were you keeping the folder then?

J: I was bringing it around with me from room to room, so it was always nearby.

T: That sounds pretty smart – this way you could record wherever the pulling started.

J: And that's what I did (opens folder and shows therapist). I pulled a few times each day during the week, all at home, and I think I got right up and wrote it down.

T: (Inspecting sheet) Looks like it was only one or two hairs per episode, which is fewer than what you told me when we first talked about this.

J: I think getting up helped me stop doing it.

T: And the information on here tells us a few other things, like the fact that you pulled during the school week when you were alone in your room and only at night – is that usually how it works?

J: I'm not too sure.

T: Well, we'll keep an eye on it to see if that's the case – we're just getting started with our detective work, so we'll have to keep watching to see if that's a regular pattern.

J: The weekend was a lot harder, though.

T: Harder in that you think you were pulling more, more stressful, or what?

J: I was really busy – I had a piano lesson first thing Saturday morning, went with my Mom to the mall Saturday afternoon, went to my friend's house Saturday night to help her babysit, then had a soccer tournament all day Sunday.

T: Wow, you had a lot going on – is that a typical weekend, or was this one especially busy?

J: No that's what they're usually like – summer's a little slower, but then I go to camp.

T: Well, I think I'm getting an idea of why the monitoring was less accurate over the weekend – seems like you were running from one place to the next. You don't have any pulling episodes down for Saturday and Sunday, but it sounds like there was some pulling –do your remember where they took place?

J: I think I pulled in the van on the way to piano, then again on the way to soccer. I also think I pulled after I got home Saturday night.

T: Were they one or two hairs each, or more?

J: More – probably at least five or ten each time.

T: Why don't we write these down on the sheet now while we're talking about them?

J: OK (takes sheet and pen).

T: I see from the school week episodes that you don't have any thoughts or feelings in the box – was there some kind of urge or itch, or was there no warning at all?

J: I guess I was tired – does that count?

T: Sure – maybe we'll find out that being tired is part of it for you. Were you tired over the weekend?

J: Yeah, I was.

T: In the mornings too?

J: Yeah, especially in the mornings.

T: How much sleep did you get Friday and Saturday night?

J: Probably about seven hours – I had to get up early both mornings.

T: Did you use an alarm clock to wake up, or did somebody wake you up?

J: Alarm clock – I set it to really loud music, because I'm not much of a morning person.

T: I ask because it looks like the pulling you remember took place on Saturday and Sunday morning, plus late Saturday night?

J: Yeah, that's right – I didn't get to bed until about 12:30 on Saturday night because my friend's parents were out pretty late and we were watching her brother.

T: So maybe being tired is something that we have to be on the lookout for.

J: Yeah.

T: Now that's really helpful – when we start putting some of the other techniques in place we may find out that being tired is a big trigger for you. We'll see how it plays out, though – some more monitoring is needed before we start drawing strong conclusions. In a lot of ways self-monitoring is like the work that the scientists in the Midwest are doing with tornado tracking – they're trying to monitor the atmosphere really carefully so that they learn as much as possible about when a tornado is forming, so they can let people in the area know as soon as possible so they can take precautions. Make sense?

J: Yeah – I think I saw a movie about that stuff a few years ago.

T: I also want to draw your attention to something else, which is that you think the episodes were a lot shorter on the days you were doing the monitoring compared to the weekend – what do you make of that?

J: Maybe getting up to go write it down stops the pulling, at least for a while?

T: Could be – we'll know more about that with time, and especially once we figure out how to make it easier to monitor when you're running all over the place on the weekends.

J: I guess I could bring it with me in the car – everybody in my family knows that I'm coming here so nobody's going to care.

T: Do you have those seat pockets in your van?

J: We do, but they're both filled with my brother's junk.

T: But they can be cleaned out pretty easily?

J: Yeah, I can do that.

T: Good – that will let you bring the folder around with you, which will make it easier to record stuff and also serve as a reminder if it's sticking out a little bit from the seat pocket in front of you.

J: Maybe I could hold it instead, since that means my hands will be doing something else.

T: That's really clever – sounds like a really good plan. We'll be doing a lot more of that kind of stuff in the weeks to come – it's great that you came up with that one yourself – it shows me that you're really thinking hard about how to outfox this trich thing.

J: Well I really want to have eyebrows and eyelashes for when I go to camp.

T: And thinking hard about trich, and monitoring as accurately as you can, will really help you to accomplish that goal – great job!

Self-monitoring difficulties of other kinds can sometimes arise, and again we emphasize the importance of the clinician taking a functional analytic approach to addressing such problems. We also suggest that therapists make every effort to collaborate with the patient in generating solutions to the problems, such as was demonstrated above. Very young children often do not have the ability to monitor their own behavior very carefully, and we suggest that parents play a more active role in keeping track of pulling behaviors with these patients. We discuss in the subsequent chapter on family issues how to encourage parental participation in monitoring TTM in young patients.

SELF-MONITORING IS AN ONGOING PROCESS

Self-monitoring continues throughout the entire protocol, since changing the contingencies in response to observed patterns can sometimes lead to changes in the pulling pattern that must themselves be monitored and addressed. An analogy we use to underscore the need to persist with monitoring because of changes in the pattern that occur in response to intervention strategies being put into place is that of trying to get rid of mice in your home: you may plug up the most obvious holes first, then find that the mice are sufficiently clever to find new holes that must then subsequently be identified and sealed. It does not mean that the plugging of the initial holes was futile, only that it was a first step that must then be followed by additional observations and actions. We use this analogy to assuage potential frustration with changes in the pulling pattern that may lead to impatience with the process and demoralization with the treatment.

OTHER FORMS OF AWARENESS TRAINING

Warning Signs. Once self-monitoring has yielded information about the context in which pulling usually occurs, another awareness training method can be incorporated into the treatment package, which is the use of visual cues in the form of warning signs. Such signs can be quite transparent, such as the words "No Pulling Zone" or a big red stop sign in a child's room, or they can be more subtle if they are to be displayed in more public areas in which the patient is concerned about other people learning about their pulling. We often use "codes" for pulling, which can vary from a hand with a slash through it, a picture of a hat or, in the case of one of our adult patients, the numbers 312.39, which is the DSM-IV-TR code for TTM. These signs should be placed in full view when possible, and can serve to improve awareness and prompt patients later on in the treatment to use their other techniques in high-risk situations. The signs themselves can also serve a stimulus control function, such as a patient who put her "no pulling" sign right in the middle of the mirror in her bedroom – because mirrors served as a trigger for her pulling, the sign both reminded her to be aware of TTM and prevented any inadvertent visual cues that could begin the chain of pulling.

Olfactory Cues. We have also found it helpful for some patients to use olfactory cues to improve their awareness of where their hand are in space; this is more likely to be helpful for those patients whose pulling of scalp hair, eyelashes, or eyebrows often begins outside of their conscious awareness. With these patients we have suggested strong perfumes, scented soaps or lotions, or other kinds of strong smells on the hands or wrists that will serve as a reminder when their hands are above their shoulders, which for many patients serves as a precursor to pulling. Those who play with the hair before pulling may find this especially useful.

Sound. In a similar vein, sounds can sometimes be used to increase patient awareness that their hand is close to their heads. Jangly bracelets are especially useful in this regard, and some of our patients who are sensitive to strong odors prefer this method instead. In a novel variation on this theme, one group of researchers modified a two-piece hearing aid by placing one piece on the patient's collar and the other on her wrist, creating a feedback noise when the patient raised her hand to her head (Rapp, Miltenberger, & Long, 1998).

CHAPTER 8

SPEED BUMPS:

Stimulus Control

Stimulus control (SC), along with competing response training and self-monitoring, is, in our opinion, one of the critical elements of cognitive behavioral therapy for most patients with TTM. Recall from Chapter 2 that TTM becomes associated over time with a variety of internal and external cues through classical conditioning (Azrin & Nunn, 1973; Mansueto et al., 1997). Simply stated, if one engages in a behavior repeatedly in a certain context, over time that context begins to elicit the behavior. For example, if one frequently snacks on potato chips while sitting on the couch and watching television, one might well find (as the authors of this book do) that one becomes hungrier as soon as the TV is turned on. A habit has been created that is partly dependent on its environmental context. Controlling the habit, therefore, may depend partly on controlling the context in which it occurs. In other words, by placing oneself in a different situation, or by changing the environment in some meaningful way, it becomes easier to control the problem behavior. Stimulus control has been used independently and as part of multi-component behavioral interventions for such diverse problems as obesity (Hall & Hall, 1982; Stuart, 1971), study skills (Fox, 1962), and health maintenance (Mayer & Frederiksen, 1986; Meyers, Thackwray, Johnson, & Schleser, 1983), although its specific efficacy with TTM is not yet well known. The incremental efficacy of SC is been established in the treatment of obesity, in which the addition of SC to other forms of behavior therapy significantly improved long-term outcome (Carroll & Yates, 1981). In surveys of adult patients receiving a multi-component group CBT for TTM, as well as child and adolescent patients receiving a similar treatment delivered in an individual format, patients rated SC as one of the most helpful components of the treatment (Brady, Diefenbach, Tolin, Hannan, & Crocetto, 2005; Tolin, Franklin, & Diefenbach, 2002).

In the case of TTM, it is important to recognize the role of two different sets of contextual stimuli: internal and external. Internal cues for pulling may include hypo-or hyper-arousal, physiological sensations, or negative cognitions (Christenson et al., 1993; Gluhoski, 1995; Mansueto, 1990). Each person's behavior is different, and is controlled by a different set of cues. Therefore, we do not automatically assume that simply because one is pulling their hair, that they are experiencing negative emotions or cognitions. Rather, we rely on a comprehensive assessment (see Chapter 4) to identify cues that are consistently associated with the problem behavior. If internal contextual cues are identified, it may be useful to consider strategies such as relaxation training or cognitive restructuring, which will be discussed later in this book. For the present Chapter, we will focus most of our attention on the control of *external* cues, as these are often clearer and easier to modify than internal cues.

External cues for pulling may include (but are not limited to) the following:

Visual Cues: People with TTM often report that their pulling is preceded by a visual scan of that region of the body. For example, a person with TTM may look at their hair in a mirror, searching for a hair that stands out in some way (e.g., is gray, shorter than the others, or curly).

Tactile/Proprioceptive Cues: Tactile cues (e.g., sensations on the skin, such as the fingertips) or proprioceptive cues (e.g., posture, placement of the hands) may also trigger urges to pull in the same manner that visual cues can. For example, prior to pulling, a person with TTM may run their fingers through their hair, searching for hair that feels different (e.g., shorter, coarser, curly). Some patients report that this behavior is pleasurable in and of itself, suggesting that pre-pulling behavior may itself be positively reinforced. Other patients have told us that pulling episodes often occur when they are sitting in a position with the hand close to the site of pulling, such as leaning the head on the left hand while driving.

Location Cues: Pulling can also be triggered when the person is a specific location. During self-monitoring, it is important to identify the places in which the problem behavior usually occurs. Some patients pull exclusively in one area of the house, for example; others may pull in a variety of locations, but the behavior is worse in certain places. We have spoken with a number of patients who report that the majority of their pulling takes place in their bedroom, while lying in bed; others are likely to pull while sitting on the living room couch; still others tend to pull in front of the bathroom mirror or while standing in the shower.

Activity Cues: Pulling can also become associated with specific activities. We often find that such activities contribute to hypo-or hyperarousal. Many of our young patients, for example, report pulling while studying or doing other forms of homework that they find stressful. Patients also often report pulling during tasks in which they feel impatient, for example, when placed on hold on the telephone, or while waiting for e-mails or instant messages on the computer. Other patients tend to pull when they are understimulated, such as while watching television or lying in bed, drifting off to sleep.

Discriminative Cues: The role of any of the above contextual cues may be modified by the presence of certain discriminative cues (factors that increase or decrease the likelihood of pulling). Thus, it is not sufficient to note that the patient typically pulls while watching television; the therapist must also ascertain the conditions under which this relationship is observed. For example, the patient may report that they pull in front of the television, but only when they are alone (i.e., the presence of others inhibits the relationship between TV watching and pulling). Another patient may pull in front of the bathroom mirror, but only when tweezers are available (i.e., the bathroom mirror is a trigger for pulling only when combined with the availability of tweezers). Thus, more subtle stimuli can either facilitate or inhibit the tendency for contextual cues to trigger pulling.

The general principle of SC is to minimize the person's exposure to stimuli that tend to trigger pulling, while maximizing their exposure to stimuli that tend to minimize pulling. This is a simple principle, although its implementation is often quite complicated and requires creative solutions. Below, we describe some SC strategies that we had used to counteract the influence of the triggering stimuli described earlier.

Visual Cues: For patients who report that their pulling is triggered by visual cues such as the sight of an irregular hair, intervention typically involves limiting the person's visual access to the area. A person who pulls hair from their scalp, eyelashes, or eyebrows while looking in the mirror might be encouraged to cover their bathroom mirror with newspaper, or, when looking in the mirror is necessary (such as when shaving or grooming), to use dim light such as candlelight in order to reduce visual acuity. A patient who pulls pubic hair while sitting on the toilet might be encouraged to drape a towel over her lap for the same reason. A patient who pulls hair from her legs or arms might be encouraged to wear long pants or long sleeves.

Tactile/Proprioceptive Cues: We frequently recommend that patients reduce tactile triggers by limiting the touching of their hair or skin. For example, we might discourage a person with TTM from playing with his hair. Often, we will encourage patients to wear rubber fingertips or gloves on one or both hands, particularly in "high risk" situations such as watching TV. These interventions have the added benefit of reducing the person's ability to pull by reducing manual dexterity. To counteract proprioceptive triggers, we will often encourage people to change positions, such as not resting their head in their hands while reading, driving, or watching TV.

Location Cues: Sometimes it is possible for the person to avoid high risk locations altogether. For example, a patient who pulls while watching TV in the basement might be encouraged to watch TV in the family living room instead; a patient who pulls in front of the bathroom mirror might be encouraged to perform her daily grooming tasks in front of a mirror in the hallway. At other times, however, avoiding these locations is not practical. In such cases, we often introduce other forms of SC into these locations to minimize the risk of pulling. For example, a patient who pulls while lying in bed might be encouraged to wear gloves to bed for this reason.

Activity Cues: Similarly, although some pulling-related activities can be avoided, others cannot. We have, at times, encouraged young people to take a break from using instant-messaging software when such activity (particularly waiting for a reply) is strongly associated with pulling. However, pulling is often associated with activities that are rewarding or otherwise integral to the person's life, and prolonged abstinence from these activities may not be possible or desirable. Therefore, to the extent possible, we find it helpful to use gloves or other tactile sensation-reducing articles, or to introduce negative discriminative cues such as those described below.

Discriminative Cues: Often, it is the little things that matter most. In many cases, the patient cannot or will not avoid high-risk situations altogether; in such cases, the therapist may introduce contextual cues that modify the relationship between the situation and the behavior. For many patients, pulling occurs only in private, when the person knows he/she will not be observed. Therefore, introducing the presence (or potential presence) of others may be a useful intervention. For example, an adolescent TTM patient may not be able to avoid lying in her bed at night, but she may be persuaded to leave her bedroom door open in order to make the situation less private. Another patient may be willing to leave the bathroom door open while shaving or putting on makeup. Often, these subtle changes in the environmental context are enough to reduce the likelihood of pulling. Some patients benefit from visual reminders, left in high-risk areas, not to pull or pick. Children in particular often enjoy making large "stop" signs to hang in the bedroom or bathroom, or by the computer or television. Other patients find it helpful to wear a brightly colored bandage on their hand or finger. This not only serves as a reminder not to pull, but also draws the unfocused puller's attention to his/her hand. An interesting variation of this principle comes from Rapp et al. (1998) who developed an "awareness enhancement device," a modified hearing aid with the earpiece worn on the wrist and the receiver attached to the collar of the shirt. This device produced a tone whenever the hand was brought within 6 in. of the collar. This device reduced hair pulling in one mentally retarded adult (Rapp et al., 1998), and thumb sucking in two children (Stricker, Miltenberger, Garlinghouse, Deaver, & Anderson, 2001).

As described in Chapter 4, pulling is usually part of a chain of stimuli and responses. During the comprehensive assessment, each part of the chain is elucidated. When implementing SC procedures, it is important to identify the earliest possible point in the chain for intervention. The most common mistake in SC (as well as competing response training and other interventions described in this book) is to wait until the last minute to implement them. By this point, the urge often has grown too strong for the person to manage. Masters, Burish, Hollon, and Rimm (1987) make this point nicely: "Self-control procedures are most easily implemented early in a response chain . . . Certain people seem to believe that the mark of self-control is the ability to withstand any and all temptation. In fact, it is far more correct to say that the mark of self-control is the ability to minimize temptation by early interruption of such behavioral chains" (pp. 451–452).

TRANSCRIPT OF SC SESSIONS

To illustrate the implementation of SC, we return to our fictitious patients from Chapter 4, Claudia and Howard. To set up the SC procedure, the therapist referred to the functional analyses diagrammed in Figures 1 and 2 of Chapter 4. We will begin by showing the conversation with Claudia.

T: OK, Claudia, you've told me a bunch about your hair pulling and how it usually goes. Let me see if I have it right. Usually, when you pull, you're studying at the desk in your room, with the door closed, and a lot of noise going on in the house.

C: Right.

T: Perhaps this would be a good place for us to start. It seems like what has happened is that you've pulled so often in that situation, that the situation itself can start to trigger urges to pull.

C: Maybe, but I don't always feel an urge to pull when I'm sitting there. The urge comes later.

T: You're right; you don't start to really feel the urge until you start stroking your hair and find a really good one, right?

C: Right. Would it make more sense for us to do something about that part of the problem?

T: I think we should do something about both parts of the problem. You see, once you start to really notice the urge, it's gotten really strong and so it would be harder for you to do something about it then. Maybe, in this situation, your best strategy would be to act early, maybe even before you start to notice the urges. It's a little bit like when you play soccer. The goalie's job is to keep the ball out of the net, right?

C: Yeah, but she doesn't always succeed.

T: Exactly. So if you're the coach, what's the best way to make sure the other team doesn't score any points?

C: Well, I guess the best strategy is to make sure they don't get the ball anywhere near the net, so the other players can take care of it.

T: Right again! In fact, your team will probably do best if you don't let the other team even get onto your half of the field!

C: You're right. I play soccer and I know that when the other team scores a goal, you can't really blame the goalie. The whole team is responsible.

T: You bet. So good defense takes place not just at the goal, when things are down to the wire, but earlier, before the other team has really started to advance. Fighting hair pulling is kind of like that. When you're really feeling the urge, and you have a good hair between your fingertips, the ball is already down by the net. At that point, it's going to be pretty hard to stop trich from doing what it wants to do.

C: So what I need to do is to take action before it gets to that point, and then my chances are better?

T: Now you've got the idea. So let's think of some things that might help while you're studying. Anyone ever come into the room while you're studying at your desk, or stroking your hair, or even pulling?

C: Sometimes my mom or my little brother will come in to bug me. They've never come in while I was pulling, but they have come in while I was stroking my hair.

T: What happened when they came in?

C: I took my hand out of my hair right away. I didn't want them to see me doing it.

T: So when other people are around, you don't do it as much?

C: No, I don't. Are you saying that should invite everybody into my room while I'm studying? I wouldn't get anything done!

T: (Laughs) No, I agree that it would be pretty tough to study with a bunch of people in your room. But what would happen if you left your bedroom door open?

C: Well, I guess I would worry that someone would see me pulling.

T: And what would be the result of that?

C: I probably wouldn't pull. But it's so noisy in the house, I need to keep the door closed.

T: What if there was another way? For example, what if we talked to your mom to see if there could be some special quiet time during the evening so you can study?

C: (Laughs) Only if they ship my brother off to Timbuktu . . .

T: (Laughs) Well, I'm not sure they could do that, but what if they sent your brother out to play in the yard for an hour, or kept him downstairs in the living room? Would that give you enough peace and quiet to study?

C: It might. I guess it's worth a try.

T: Great! We've got something we can try. Now the other part of this is that while you're studying, you sit like this (rests had in hand, touching hair with fingertips). What do you think about that?

C: I suppose it makes it easier for me to start pulling.

T: Yes, and it also makes it more likely that you'll find a really good hair with your fingers, and then . . .

C: Whammo.

T: Right. So what would be a good solution?

C: I guess maybe I shouldn't sit like that.

T: Maybe not. How else could you sit?

C: I guess I could put my hands on the desk in front of me, or maybe hold onto my book. Maybe I could even sit on my hands, or put my hands in my pockets.

T: Great ideas! Now, how about something to help you remember not to pull?

C: You mean, like a sign or something?

T: Something like that. What do you think would work for you?

C: I guess I could make a big stop sign on my computer, you know, something in bright red, and tape it to the computer screen.

T: That sounds like a terrific idea.

C: You know, now that I'm thinking about it, maybe I could change my screen-saver on my computer to say, "Don't pull."

T: Very creative! I think you're on your way.

As you may recall from Chapter 4, Howard's hair pulling did not follow the same pattern as did Claudia's hair pulling. Therefore, he requires a slightly different set of interventions. Howard's transcript is below.

T: I think I'm getting a pretty good sense of how your hair pulling goes. If I under-stand it right, mostly this happens when you're sitting in your reclining chair, watching TV by yourself.

H: That's right. I really don't do it anywhere else.

T: And you were saying that is usually no one else in the room, right? Your wife is in the kitchen or maybe in her sewing room, and the kids are out in the yard.

H: Definitely. I'd be really embarrassed if anyone saw me do it.

T: What happens when they're in the room?

H: Then I just don't do it. I don't even want to.

T: And you're usually <u>not even aware that you're doing it</u>, right? You're just sitting there in the chair, with your legs up, feeling kind of bored and sleepy, and the next thing you know, you've done it.

H: Right. I don't even know it's happened until it's over.

T: So there's a tricky issue here. It's hard to imagine how you can stop pulling, if you don't even know you're doing it. But maybe there's another way. When you pull again and again, in the same situation, doing the same activities, over time all of those elements – the TV, the chair, your position, feeling sleepy – all become associated with pulling. When I watch TV, I like to eat potato chips. I know it's a bad habit, but what can you do? I'm used to it. <u>It's become a habit.</u> So now I decide that I need to lose some weight, and so I want to go on a diet. So I tell myself, "no more potato chips." I do pretty well until Sunday, when the football game comes on. I sit down in front of the TV, and what happens?

H: You want potato chips and your diet goes out the window.

T: Exactly. You see how that happens? I eat potato chips over and over again in front of the TV, until eventually . . .

H: Just being in front of the TV makes you want to eat potato chips.

T: Right. So if I want to stop eating those chips . . .

H: You have to stop watching TV?

T: Well, that would be one option. But I like watching TV, and I'd hate to miss the football game.

H: So maybe you just have to do something different. Like not have any potato chips in the house. Or maybe you have to have your wife watch the game with you, so she can stop you from eating.

T: You've definitely got the idea! If you want to control the problem, one of the very best ways is to figure out what kinds of situations are "high risk" for you, and then try to change that situation in some way.

H: Watching TV in my recliner is definitely a high-risk situation for me.

T: OK, so knowing that, what could you do about it?

H: Well, I'm like you; I don't want to give up TV. But maybe if my wife or my kids were in the room with me, I wouldn't want to pull.

T: So one thing you could do would be to limit your TV watching to times when other people are in the room.

H: I could do that some of the time, like in the evening. But the rest of my family doesn't like to watch football, and I doubt that they want to be in there with me.

T: So we have to get a little more creative. You usually pull from your legs, right?

H: Right . . .Hey, maybe if I just wore long pants instead of shorts, it would be harder for me to get at those hairs.

T: It certainly seems like that might help. How about your posture? Do you think it would help if you didn't recline in the chair?

H: Well, it wouldn't make any harder for me to reach my knee . . . but it might make me feel less sleepy. In fact, maybe it would help if I just brought in a different chair to sit in, maybe one that isn't quite so comfortable.

T: Great idea.

CHAPTER 9

ACTIVE STRATEGIES FOR ACTIVE HANDS:

Competing Response Training

In this chapter, we review one of the more commonly used components of CBT for TTM, competing response training (CRT). Azrin and Nunn (1973) introduced CRT as a component of habit reversal training (HRT), a general intervention for nervous habits and tics. The original HRT was a multi-component intervention that included self-monitoring, awareness training, motivational enhancement, and competing response practice. The other elements of HRT are described in other chapters in this book. In this chapter, we will focus on the competing response training aspect of HRT in this chapter.

Azrin and Nunn's original rationale for HRT posited that nervous habits persist partly because they operate outside conscious awareness, and, in some cases, because the muscles used to perform the nervous habit have become overdeveloped compared to the opposing muscle groups. This rationale seems to fit TTM and other body-focused impulse control disorders only partially. As described earlier in this book, these behaviors sometimes take place outside of awareness (e.g., unfocused pulling); however, in many cases the person is quite aware of the behavior. Furthermore, there is no evidence at this time to suggest that the muscles used for pulling become overdeveloped, or that opposing muscle groups become underdeveloped. CRT is also based partially on the principle of "overcorrection," conceptualized as a relatively mild form of punishment. Originally, overcorrection involved enforcing a behavior or set of behaviors that corrects or is the "opposite" of the problem behavior (Azrin, Kaplan, & Foxx, 1973; Foxx & Azrin, 1972).

Overcorrection involved interrupting problem behavior, physically guiding (or forcing) the individual through a behavior that corrects any negative outcomes from the problem act and perhaps serves as a desirable alternative, and requiring the individual to engage in repeated, exaggerated practice of this new behavior. Thus, overcorrection included negative contingencies for undesired behavior, combined with positive practice of opposing behavior.

Matson, Stephens, and Smith (1978) demonstrated the potential of over-correction for hair pulling in the treatment of an institutionalized mentally retarded woman. In this case, the woman was instructed to brush her hair for 10 minutes every time she pulled a hair. The frequency of hair pulling was reduced dramatically within three days, and was nearly eliminated after 42 days of treatment. Treatment gains were maintained over a three-month follow-up period. Barrett and Shapiro (1980) found similar results in their treatment of an institutionalized mentally retarded young girl. When this girl was required to brush her hair for two minutes after each hair-pulling episode that occurred during her classes, the frequency of hair pulling decreased substantially: the behavior was eliminated after 24 interventions over 12 days. When the treatment was withdrawn, the girl's hair-pulling increased in frequency; however, when overcorrection was applied in her residential unit as well as in her classroom, more stable results were obtained and the girl was no longer pulling hair at 12-month follow-up.

In their translation of overcorrection to CRT, Azrin and Nunn (1973) eliminated the punitive elements of overcorrection. Specifically, patients were not required to provide "restitution" for their actions, nor were they physically forced to engage in competing responses. Furthermore, CRT provided a potentially more desirable intervention than overcorrection, as it could be applied *before* the behavior began. In CRT, patients were trained to perform an opposing movement whenever they felt the urge to engage in their nervous habits. Positive practice of these movements was accomplished by encouraging patients to engage in the behavior frequently, and for a prolonged period of time (approximately three minutes). In a case series of 12 patients with a variety of nervous habits and tics, a specific opposing movement was developed for each patient. A patient with a tic that involved jerking the shoulder upward, for example, was taught to draw his shoulders downward and hold them there. A patient who pulled her eyelashes was taught to grasp objects firmly in her hands whenever she felt the urge to pull. Another patient who bit his fingernails received a similar intervention. Of the 12 patients, 11 showed virtual elimination of their habits. In a follow-up study (Azrin, Nunn, & Frantz-Renshaw, 1982), a single session of HRT with CRT proved superior to a single session of negative practice, in which patients with unwanted oral habits were instructed to engage in the undesired behavior for a prolonged period of time. Intriguingly, this single session of HRT resulted in a 99% reduction of the behavior over a 22-month follow-up.

Having tried HRT with one TTM patient in the study described above, Azrin et al. (1980) randomly assigned 34 TTM patients to either HRT (which included CRT, self-monitoring, inconvenience review, social support, and awareness training) or negative practice (in which they were asked to go through the motions of hair-pulling, without actually pulling hair, for 30 seconds every hour). Although patients in both conditions reported a decrease in the frequency of pulling, the patients who received HRT with CRT showed a much stronger and more durable response. In four case studies of CRT with patients with relatively mild TTM (Rosenbaum & Ayllon, 1981), patients were instructed to place their hands in their lap or at their sides, and to clench their fists for 2 minutes, at the first sign of urges to pull, if they noticed themselves beginning to pull, or if they actually pulled. To facilitate generalization outside of the therapy session, patients were also instructed to practice the competing response while imagining themselves in a high-risk situation. Hair pulling was eliminated in all four subjects, and remained at zero through a 6-month follow-up period. Tarnowski and colleagues (1987) used HRT with CRT to treat hair-pulling in a young girl with severe TTM. This girl was unable to self-monitor; therefore, treatment outcome was assessed using visual analysis of alopecia. Results indicated substantial hair regrowth.

As described above, the original HRT protocol was a multi-component intervention that featured CRT but also included awareness training, self-monitoring, motivational procedures, and generalization procedures. Thus, it is difficult to use these studies to determine the specific efficacy of CRT. In an early dismantling study, Ladoceur (1979) assigned 50 patients with unwanted nail-biting behaviors to one of five conditions: habit reversal (in this case, awareness training and CRT), habit reversal plus self-monitoring, self-monitoring alone, self-monitoring plus daily graph plotting, or waitlist. Results indicated that the four treated groups improved significantly more than did the waitlist group; however, there were no significant differences among the groups. Ladoceur suggested that the active ingredient in HRT might be an increase in awareness of the problem behavior, rather than learning a competing response. More recently, Woods, Miltenberger, and Lumley (1996) reported that awareness training and self-monitoring were sufficient to reduce motor tics in two of four children, suggesting that at least some patients may benefit from enhanced awareness alone, without requiring training in competing responses. The remaining two children, who did not respond to awareness training and self-monitoring alone, responded to the addition of CRT, suggesting that CRT may yield benefits over and above heightened awareness.

Subsequent researchers (e.g., Miltenberger, Fuqua, & McKinley, 1985) have abbreviated and simplified the HRT protocol to focus on awareness training (see Chapter 7) and CRT. This simpler protocol was used in the successful treatment of three adolescents with TTM (Rapp, Miltenberger, Long, Elliott, & Lumley, 1998). Three to four competing responses (e.g., folding arms, sitting on hands) were selected for each child, and the child was encouraged to engage in one of these behaviors every time they pulled or felt the urge to pull. Two of the children showed substantial reductions in the frequency of hair pulling, although "booster" sessions were required to prevent relapse. The third child showed an initial reduction in hair pulling, but appeared to relapse and discontinued treatment. The applicability of simplified HRT with CRT to skin picking was demonstrated in a case report of two brothers with this disorder (Twohig & Woods, 2001b). In each case, the patient was instructed to make a closed fist for one minute whenever he picked his skin or engaged in a pre-picking behavior (e.g., rubbing his skin). Results indicated that although skin picking was not eliminated, the frequency of the behavior was reduced substantially from baseline.

In clinical practice, CRT training often involves encouraging patients to touch, squeeze, or play with objects when they feel an urge to pull. Patients with TTM often like to play with a rubber "koosh" ball, perhaps because of the hair-like quality of the rubber "legs." We therefore encourage patients to keep these toys handy wherever and whenever they perceive as high risk for pulling. A patient, therefore, might be encouraged to buy several "koosh" balls and place one in their car, next to their bed, by the sofa, etc. They would be instructed to pick up one of these toys whenever they felt an urge to pull. Over time, the patient is taught to pick up the toy progressively earlier in the pulling sequence. Eventually, patients learn to engage in the opposing behavior before they are conscious of urges to pull but recognize the situation as "high risk."

There is virtually no limit to the number of possible CRT behaviors. What is critical is that the behavior is (a) easy for the person to implement, and (b) motorically inconsistent with pulling. CRT activities we have used include:

- playing with clay
- playing "cat's cradle" with a ball of string
- shelling peanuts
- tying and retying one's shoes
- playing with jewelry, such as a ring, necklace, or bracelet
- squeezing a "stress ball"
- in classroom settings, squeezing a book or pencil
- squeezing the steering wheel of the car

CRT does not necessarily require that the person have something to hold in their hands. Examples of possible "self-contained" CRT behaviors include:

- making a fist and squeezing
- putting one's hands into one's pockets
- sitting on one's hands

Additional CRT activities are shown in the patient handout (see Appendix).

Following the principle of overcorrection, we generally recommend that patients engage in the competing behavior for 3 full minutes. However, our experience has been that many patients have difficulty complying with this instruction; therefore, we often modify our instructions to engage in the competing behavior for 1 minute, or as little as 30 seconds for children and adolescents. The long-duration competing response is not done for punitive reasons, as might be said of overcorrection. Rather, the 3-minute duration is designed to allow the person's urge to pull to subside while they are doing the competing behavior; briefer durations may not be successful (Twohig & Woods, 2001a). In this manner, we conceptualize CRT as being somewhat akin to the response prevention element of CBT for obsessive-compulsive disorder (Kozak & Foa, 1997). Over time, the patient has learned that the best (and perhaps only) way to reduce their feelings of internal discomfort is to engage in the compulsive/impulsive behavior. Response prevention and CRT demonstrate to patients that if they do not pull, their discomfort will subside anyway, although not as quickly. Thus, in addition to the behavioral aspect of training a competing behavior, from a cognitive perspective, CRT teaches patients that they do not need to pull in order to reduce discomfort.

TRANSCRIPT OF CRT SESSION

Daniel is a 26-year old man who has been diagnosed with TTM. Functional analysis (see Chapter 4) indicated that Daniel tends to pull while watching TV and when looking in the bathroom mirror for grooming purposes. Pulling is lessened, but not eliminated, when others are in the room. His pre-pulling behaviors involve stroking the hair on his scalp until he identifies a hair that is shorter, curlier, or coarser than the others. Once he has found the hair, he feels a strong urge to pull it. After pulling the hair, he tends to roll it between his fingers, inspect the root visually, and occasionally rub the hair across his lips. He reports a feeling of decreased tension and increased satisfaction after pulling.

In this session, the therapist (T) introduces the concept of CRT to Daniel (D), and provides him with introductory exercises. Note that initially, the aim is simply to get Daniel used to the exercise, rather than to prevent pulling.

T: Daniel, in our previous sessions we've discussed how your hair pulling usually goes, and I think I have a pretty good idea of not only how you pull, but what kinds of situations tend to make you want to pull, as well as what you get out of pulling. We've also worked on some ways to increase your own awareness of pulling, such as where your hands are, what your fingers are doing, and so on. Now let's start to work on reducing the pulling itself.

D: Sounds good. I really want to get this under control.

T: Great. What I'm going to suggest to you might seem a little strange, and it might be kind of inconvenient for you. But bear with me for a moment, because this is the best way we know of to help people stop pulling. Basically, I'm going to ask you to do something else with your hands whenever you find yourself pulling. We can pick any activity we want, as long as it meets certain criteria. It has to be something that you can do easily, without needing a lot of preparation. It also has to be something that you can sustain for three minutes. It also has to be something that would physically prevent you from pulling—meaning you couldn't possibly pull hair while doing it. Finally, it has to be something that you'd feel comfortable doing when other people are around, because you often pull when others are in the room with you. Any ideas?

D: Boy, that's a toughie. I guess if I knew of something else to do with my hands, I would have done it already. I've tried things like playing with a stress ball; that really didn't work for me.

T: I see. So it's kind of hard for you to see how this could work now.

D: Right.

T: When you tried using the stress ball before, how did you do it?

D: Well, I would just go get it when I felt like pulling, and then I'd just play around with it for a few seconds. But a lot of the time I found that I would start pulling while I was looking for the ball! And even if I could hold out until I found the ball, it seemed like I'd just start pulling again once I put it down.

T: Okay, so there were a couple of things about that plan that weren't working for you. One was that you had to go looking for the ball, and you'd sometimes start pulling during that process. The other was that the pulling would just start up again when you stopped playing with the ball. Is that right?

D: Yeah, that's it.

T: So perhaps we could make that work better by changing a couple of things. First we have the fact that searching for the ball isn't helping. So how could we fix that?

D: I guess I could keep the ball in my pocket. It's pretty small so I could do that.

T: Great idea. But I know that sometimes you pull in the bathroom, right when you get out of the shower. I assume you aren't wearing pants in there!

D: (Laughs) No. Well, I have a couple of those stress balls—maybe I could just keep one on the bathroom counter.

T: That sounds like a good plan. So maybe by having the stress balls within reach all the time, we'll take care of that part of it. But now we have this other part— in your experience, you start pulling as soon as you put the stress ball down. There are a couple of things you told me about how you use the ball that give me some clues about how we could improve that. You said that you would just kind of play around with the ball—what would you do, exactly?

D: I'd just, you know, hold it, maybe give it a squeeze or two.

T: So perhaps we could change that up by having you squeeze the ball right from the start and hold onto it really tightly the whole time, like you're trying to fatigue the muscles of your hand. The other thing you said was that you would only play with the ball for a few seconds. How about if we increase that, and have you squeeze the ball for three whole minutes?

D: Well, I get the part about squeezing the ball; that makes sense. But why three minutes? That seems like an awfully long time.

T: Yes, it is a long time. That's part of what may be helpful about it. You see, often, beating urges to pull doesn't necessarily mean that you have to be 100% free of the urges, 100% of the time. In many cases, all you really need is to be able to get through that immediate period when the urges are really strong. By squeezing the stress ball for three minutes, what you're doing is making sure that you're squeezing long enough for the urge to come down to a level where you can resist it. You're also doing something else: You're showing yourself that you don't need to pull in order for your urges to get better; if you hang in there and do something else besides pulling, you'll see that your urges can come down anyway.

D: Okay, I get it. But what happens if I get another urge after the three minutes?

T: My hope is that after three minutes, your urges will feel a lot more controllable. But if you get another urge, then you would just squeeze the ball again for another three minutes.

D: Okay, I guess I'm willing to try just about anything.

T: Great. Let me show you how it will go. (Takes a stress ball from the desk drawer and places it on the desk) I have my stress ball here, on the bathroom counter, just like we agreed. Now I'll start shaving, just like you do (mimics shaving). Now, I start looking at my hair in the mirror, and my hand goes up to my head (starts playing with hair). I find a hair that feels kind of course, one that I'd really like to pull. (Removes hand from hair and picks up stress ball with the same hand) So now I drop what I'm doing, grab the stress ball, and squeeze. And I'll hold it that way for three minutes. Now you try it. (Places the stress ball in front of Daniel). Start pretending to shave.

D: This feels a little goofy.

T: I know; it is a little goofy! But you can see that I'm willing to be goofy right along with you. And maybe if we can both be a little goofy here, we'll get you into a better position to beat trich.

D: Okay, I guess I've got nothing to lose. (Mimics shaving)

T: That's good. Now, look in the mirror and see that hair. Put your hand up there and feel around until you find a really good, coarse hair. (Daniel does so). Very good. What are you experiencing right now?

D: I'd like to pull it.

T: Perfect. On a scale from 0–10, how strong is that urge to pull?

D: About an 8.

T: Okay. Now, quickly, drop your hand away from your head and grab the stress ball. Squeeze it nice and hard—not so hard that you hurt your hand, but hard enough that it would make your hand muscles start to get tired. (Daniel does so). Now let's look at the clock and wait for three minutes to go by. (Both wait for three minutes) Excellent; you can put the ball down now. On a scale from 0–10, how strong is your urge to pull hair right now?

D: Maybe a 2.

T: So you see, your urge can come down even if you don't pull hair—you can wait it out and just stay on top of the urge, without giving in to it, and it will eventually decrease.

Next, the therapist accompanied Daniel to the clinic bathroom, where Daniel stood in front of the mirror and practiced the sequence again. The reason for this extra step was to facilitate generalization to situations outside of the therapist's office. In the next session, they also practiced the same sequence while sitting on a sofa, pretending to watch television, as this was another high-risk situation for Daniel.

Daniel's self-monitoring sheets (see Chapter 7) showed that his hair pulling frequency decreased over the next two weeks, but was not completely eliminated. The therapist used this information as a starting point for a trouble-shooting discussion.

T: It looks like you're really doing a good job with the stress ball, and your records show me that you're pulling less hair. I also see that although you've been able to reduce the hair pulling, you're still pulling some of the time—it looks like more in the bathroom now than on the couch.

D: That's right. It's great that I could get it down; that's really encouraging. But I'd be a lot happier if I could stop completely.

T: Absolutely. Let's see if we can make this even more helpful for you. Tell me a little about the times that it's working.

D: Well, the times that it's working are when I notice that I have a hold of the hair on my head and I'm about to pull it, and I can get myself to put my hand down and pick up the stress ball. Usually, if I can do that, I'm OK.

T: And the times that it's not working?

D: Well, what happens is that sometimes, when I have my hand up on my head, it seems like I just don't have enough willpower to put my hand down. It's like I'm out of control or something.

T: I think I understand. And I should tell you that in my opinion, it's not an issue of willpower—you have plenty of that. When this strategy isn't working, I think it's because there are some ways that it could be more effective, not because there's something wrong with you.

D: That's good to know. How could we make it more effective?

T: Perhaps what's happening is that you pass a "point of no return" when your hand is up to your scalp, and at that point it's just really hard for you to stop yourself.

D: That's definitely what it feels like. It's just too hard to take my hand away from my head.

T: Okay, so knowing that, what could we do differently?

D: You mean besides wear handcuffs all day (laughs)? I don't know . . .I guess maybe if I didn't let myself get to that point . . .

T: You're on to something there.

D: So are we talking about grabbing the squeeze ball before my hand gets up to my head?

T: I think that might be a very good solution for you. As we've discussed before, there's a chain of events that leads up to your pulling the hair. It probably starts when you enter the bathroom, maybe even earlier, and then gathers steam when you look in the mirror, gets even stronger when you start looking at your hair, and so on, so by the time you have that one hair between your fingertips, the train is going 100 miles an hour and it's hard to put on the brakes.

D: That really seems true. It does feel like a train picking up speed.

T: And so the best way to stop the train may be to catch it while it's still moving slow, just pulling out of the station. The question, then, is: When would be the best time for you to act to interrupt that chain of events?

D: What about right when I walk up to the mirror?

T: Good idea.

D: But should I do that even if I'm not having any urges to pull?

T: Yes, I think so. Because we know from your experience that, even if you aren't having an urge right then, the urge is likely to show up eventually. So let's try to nip it in the bud.

Based on this discussion, Daniel's new homework was to engage in the competing behavior at an earlier stage of the hair-pulling sequence, when he first entered the bathroom. He found that by doing so, he experienced much fewer urges to pull, and the frequency of his pulling continued to decrease.

Chapter 10

HOLDING THE LEAD:

Maintenance

We begin this section with a brief consideration of factors associated with treatment outcome and maintenance of gains over time. As we discussed in Chapter 5, the literature on long-term maintenance of gains following any treatment for TTM or other BFRBs is quite limited, but the data collected thus far suggest that relapse is apparently quite common. One factor that has emerged from the CBT outcome literature for other disorders is that the better a patient does in the short term the better off they will do in the long term (e.g., Simpson et al., 2004). This is convergent with conceptual models of OCD and other anxiety disorders that emphasize the importance of negative reinforcement: if a patient is still ritualizing and/or avoiding at the end of treatment then fear and distress associated with obsessions will be maintained. We found similar results in our study of children and adolescents with TTM (Tolin et al., 2006): of the children classified as "responders" (a clinician's rating of "much improved" or "very much improved") at post-treatment, 24% lost this designation during follow-up. However, none of the children classified as "excellent responders" (a clinician's rating of "very much improved") at post-treatment lost that designation during follow-up. Harkening back to our theoretical model of TTM that emphasizes the importance of both positive and negative reinforcement in maintaining TTM, it also follows that if urges to pull are being reinforced by pulling then the strength of those urges will be maintained; alternatively, the lower the ratio of reinforced urges over the total number of urges, the weaker the urges will be over time. Most nicotine addicts will attest to this relationship as well: the longer they go without smoking the weaker the urges to smoke become, until such time that contextual factors such as time of day (e.g., immediately after dinner), sight of others smoking, smell of cigarette smoke, and negative affective states no longer evoke the same intensity of urges previously. Similarly, we expect that TTM works in much the same way, which underscores the importance of encouraging patients to use the various techniques that comprise the core of this manual to decrease the reinforced urge:total urge ratio. Accordingly, we include in our literature summary a discussion of factors associated with post-treatment outcome as well as those associated with long-term outcome.

MAINTENANCE OF GAINS: WHAT DOES THE EMPIRICAL LITERATURE TELL US?

Below, we summarize the literature on maintenance of gains following CBT for TTM. Difficulty accruing the very large samples of patients who have entered and/or completed treatment for TTM has slowed the scientific study of predictors, and accordingly the literature is replete with inconsistent findings, null results, or studies with clear methodological problems. That said, the data thus far will be considered in our subsequent discussions of how best to maximize treatment gains and to promote maintenance over time.

As we have already mentioned, a wide array of behavioral and cognitive-behavioral treatments and treatment packages has been applied to TTM, involving components such as self-monitoring, aversion, covert sensitization, negative practice, relaxation training, habit reversal/competing response training, and overcorrection. Of these, the package that has received the most attention thus far in the literature on TTM and other habit/impulse control disorders is HRT (Azrin & Nunn, 1973), which typically includes awareness training, self monitoring procedures, and CRT. One of the difficulties in interpreting the literature on TTM outcome and maintenance of gains is that there have not been as yet any large-scale dismantling studies, so it is unclear from the outcome literature whether some treatment packages would have been better than others in reducing TTM and related dysfunction at post-treatment, and thus would have also been associated with better maintenance of gains. We have attempted in this book to distill what is known empirically and clinically about which techniques constitute the core elements of treatment and which are adjunctive, and although we have some empirical backing for our decisions based on our clinical research, nevertheless interpretation of the literature on maintenance is fraught with difficulty for these reasons.

Although successful outcomes following some of these behavioral and cognitive-behavioral interventions are reported, the vast majority of the literature consists of uncontrolled case reports or small case series (Keuthen et al., 1999). In the first randomized group study comparing behavioral treatments for TTM (Azrin et al., 1980), HR was more effective than negative practice, with patients in the HR group reporting a 99% reduction in number of hair pulling episodes compared to a 58% reduction for patients in the negative practice group. The authors report that the HR group maintained their gains at 22-month follow-up, with patients reporting 87% reduction compared to pre-treatment. The generalizability of these findings was limited by the absence of a formal treatment protocol, exclusive reliance on self-reports as the sole outcome measures, and by the fact that only a small subset of patients completed follow-ups.

Since then, three more RCTs have been published and their results converge to support CBT as an efficacious treatment for TTM. In a small trial, Ninan et al. (2000) found CBT package emphasizing HR superior to clomipramine (CMI) and PBO at post treatment; CMI and PBO failed to separate from one another. No follow-up data were available from this trial, so it is unclear whether the CBT gains were maintained over time. van Minnen et al. (2003) randomized 43 patients with TTM to receive either behavior therapy (HR), fluoxetine (FLU), or waitlist (WL) for 12 weeks. Patients in the HR group experienced a greater reduction in their TTM symptoms than did patients in the FLU or WL groups. However, these authors did report that the gains associated with their behavioral protocol were generally not stable over a two-year follow-up period (Keijsers et al., 2006). As was the case in our pediatric study (Tolin et al., 2006), post-treatment abstinence from hair-pulling was associated with better long-term maintenance.

In response to the evidence that CBT's effects do not appear to be complete and that relapse is a common problem, Woods et al. (2006) added Acceptance and Commitment Therapy (ACT) to a HR protocol. These investigators found HR/ACT superior to WL at post-treatment, although the study design did not allow for conclusions about the separate contributions of ACT and habit reversal, respectively. Those who received the combined protocol appeared to maintain their gains through a three-month follow-up period, which is encouraging and perhaps the result of having included a component purported to reduce experiential avoidance, which is apparently common in TTM (Begotka et al., 2003).

The randomized studies discussed above and several open studies of BT or CBT that have included follow-up data suggest problems with relapse in adults. Lerner et al. (1998), Keuthen et al. (2001), and Mouton and Stanley (1996) also indicated that relapse was common, whereas Azrin et al. (1980) reported maintenance of gains. It is important to note that the studies that found problems with relapse used independent assessment of TTM symptoms via semi-structured interview or a psychometrically sound self-report instrument, whereas Azrin et al's study relied on unstandardized patient self-report. Single case reports are also generally mixed on whether patients maintained their treatment gains (e.g., Friman et al., 1984). Clinically, several TTM treatment experts (e.g., Christenson & Mackenzie, 1995) have observed that patients often experience recurrence of hairpulling after treatment, especially in response to external stressors.

Stanley and Mouton (1996) suggested that additional attention might need to be given to extending awareness training and the use of competing responses to maximize long-term outcome. These data in adults led us to emphasize relapse prevention in our original pediatric TTM project, and to include maintenance and follow-up phases in our ongoing research. Given our very encouraging outcomes for children and adolescents randomized to CBT in the RCT with respect to post-treatment reduction of TTM symptoms, maintenance of gains through an eight-week maintenance phase and a six-month naturalistic follow-up phase, we encourage therapists using this manual to continue this emphasis and to include maintenance phases and regular long-term "check-ups" after treatment has been completed.

STRATEGIES FOR PREVENTING RELAPSE AND RECURRENCE

Below, we discuss a number of points that we try to underscore in order to promote maintenance of gains, and later we provide clinical examples of how to manage common difficulties that patients encounter after acute treatment has been completed. Because good post-treatment status appears to predict long-term maintenance of gains, many of the clinical strategies we use to maximize benefit during acute treatment are thought to serve the dual purpose of helping patients remain well. However, there are also several strategies that we employ specifically to address maintenance, although many of these strategies are introduced towards the end of acute treatment rather than after treatment is completed.

For this component of treatment, we borrow liberally from the research literature on relapse prevention. Originally developed for substance abuse treatment, the aims of relapse prevention are to prevent the return of symptoms, and to help patients get "back on track" if lapses occur (e.g., Parks, Anderson, & Marlatt, 2001). Although not formally tested in TTM, relapse prevention has shown promise in the treatment of other disorders such as OCD (Hiss, Foa, & Kozak, 1994; McKay, 1997; McKay, Todaro, Neziroglu, & Yaryura-Tobias, 1996). Relapse prevention strategies commonly include educating the patient about the likely precursors of relapse, a discussion of the "abstinence violation effect," in which an isolated occurrence of the problem behavior cues the patient to give up trying and to return to old habits, and making plans for continued treatment as needed. Specific applications for TTM are detailed below.

EMPHASIZE HOW PROGRESS WAS MADE IN THE FIRST PLACE

Patients who have made substantial progress in CBT for TTM or related problems often become alarmed at the prospect of having to fight TTM "on their own" once the treatment course has been completed. Here we first emphasize the booster session schedule that has typically been set up in advance (e.g., bi-monthly sessions, monthly sessions, followed by "check-ups" as needed) and that more generally we as clinicians will remain open to helping down the road. At the same time, we spend a good deal of time in later CBT sessions emphasizing to the patient who has made significant progress that they and not the therapist are ultimately responsible for the good outcome because they had the difficult task of identifying high-risk situations via careful self-monitoring, putting "speed bumps" into place with stimulus control methods, and implementing habit reversal methods at the first sign of urges to pull. We also emphasize that the patient is now, through their own hard work, much more knowledgeable about TTM, the theoretical foundation of CBT approaches, and in how best to implement the treatment procedures that flow from their new-found theoretical understanding of how TTM works in them specifically and how it should be addressed. We remind our patients that now that they have completed a course of CBT, they are more knowledgeable about these key issues than are many if not most mental health professionals: our pediatric patients in particular are often most surprised and proud of this, and we emphasize it repeatedly. Towards the end of treatment when substantial progress has been achieved, we often ask our patients to recount to us how they were able to make progress on their TTM, and quiz them on what to do if a new urge to pull that they had not encountered previously was to occur (e.g., eyelash pulling in a patient who has previously only pulled scalp hair). Patients are often able to answer such questions without difficulty, and can choose treatment strategies for the hypothetical new urges that flow logically from CBT theory. We take every opportunity we can to reinforce their new-found knowledge in order to allay concerns that the therapist, clinic, etc., was primarily responsible for the change and that relapse must necessarily follow if the contact is decreased. With younger patients we sometimes formalize this process by holding a graduation ceremony in the last session (see March & Mulle, 1998, for examples from pediatric OCD) in which we present a certificate of achievement, invite relatives, and provide refreshments – analogies to the Wizard of Oz are sometimes helpful here, where the emphasis is placed at the end of acute treatment on what the child had inside of him/her all along to fight successfully against the Wicked Witch of Trich. The similarity between completing a CBT program successfully and graduating from school is emphasized in order to reinforce the patient's achievement of mastery over the subject matter, and the need for further "self-study" to retain the knowledge can also be underscored simultaneously.

Normalize Post-treatment Urges

By the time the latter stages of acute CBT have been reached, the patient should already be quite familiar with the fact that most if not all people with TTM have at least some ongoing urges to pull or even actual pulling. Accordingly, patients who are still experiencing urges and pulling some in response to urges towards the end of treatment should be told that this is to be expected not only because the patient has a biological vulnerability to TTM but also because the habit of pulling in response to urges has been strengthened over the course of months or often years and thus TTM typically won't "give up the ship" after a relatively short intervention. For our adult patients or for pediatric patients whose parents have quit smoking at some point, an analogy to the urges to smoke is often helpful here: immediately post-quitting, most smokers still often have strong urges to smoke at times and in places where they used to smoke. However, with repeated non-reinforcement of these urges over time, the connection between environmental circumstances or affective states and smoking will gradually weaken. Simply the nature of the beast, we tell our patients, and thus nothing to be especially surprised about or worried about, provided of course that the patient is continuing to use the CBT strategies they found helpful in reducing pulling during the acute treatment. It is critically important to highlight this point, since the patient who is soon to leave treatment may be frightened by the fact that urges and some pulling are still present or, in the case where the patient has made very substantial progress, could recur. We emphasize that the presence of an urge to pull should no longer be a cause for alarm, since the treatment focused specifically on developing effective methods to deal with these urges differently and successfully. The patient should instructed to openly acknowledge the presence of urges when they occur, use the stimulus control and CRT techniques they employed during acute treatment, and allow the urges to pass of their own accord and in their own good time. We have been accused of pessimism on occasion by emphasizing the likely persistence of urges even after a very successful treatment course, but believe strongly that it is more therapeutic to prepare the patient for this likely possibility than to turn a blind eye to data about their persistence.

Discuss Lapses and Relapses

As noted above, we underscore the likely occurrence of urges even after treatment has been completed successfully. In keeping with this same spirit of preparing patients for a long-term battle against TTM, a plan should be put in place towards the end of treatment for managing significant lapses or a relapse. This plan should include psychoeducation about what to expect in the long run with respect to urges and pulling behavior, define lapses (temporary slip-ups in refraining from pulling and/or occurrence of intense urges) and relapses (a return to the old ways of managing urges to pull hair), and provide tailored instructions about what to do when the TTM is especially troublesome. We are careful at this stage to emphasize that an occasional urge to pull or even occasional pulling does not even constitute a "lapse," but is better viewed as a natural occurrence that then involves a set of choices, some of which are likely to further weaken the TTM and some of which can strengthen it. The response to a given lapse is thus emphasized over its mere occurrence, and patients should be instructed that responding by putting the treatment techniques into place is associated with better long-term outcome.

When the patient's response to urges involves a return to more than occasional pulling, this lapse should be addressed directly. As we have emphasized above with respect to TTM psychopathology, sometimes the pulling is less intentional, i.e., occurs almost automatically because of the long history of responding in this manner. If this is indeed the case, the patient should be instructed to make a note of the lapse and, if feasible, to consider whether the return to automatic or unfocused pulling being reported was predictable based on the information gathered during awareness training, i.e., occurred at a time and under environmental and affective circumstances that were identified previously as "high risk." If so, the patient should be encouraged to revisit the lapse in detail in order to determine if there were techniques used in such circumstances during acute treatment that were not implemented in this most recent lapse. For example, if the patient's last lapse occurred while surfing the web on the computer in the seclusion of the den, did they fail to put on the hat that had become a requirement for sitting in that room alone during acute treatment? When such lapses occur, the patient should be told that ignoring the lapse or catastrophizing them are *both* likely to be unhelpful, and that instead it is important to go back and simply examine what happened, consider what could be done in future similar circumstances, and to create a specific plan to be followed the next time. Patients who are experiencing frequent intentional lapses over the course of several days and find themselves abandoning the techniques previously found useful may be in the midst of a more significant relapse, and should be encouraged to recontact the therapist quickly if they are not in regular treatment at that time and to inform a supportive person in their lives that they are experiencing significant difficulty. We emphasize that one or even an occasional lapse does not constitute a relapse, since patients often become hypervigilant about this issue after treatment has been completed.

ENCOURAGE LIFESTYLE ADJUSTMENTS

As we now know from a large-scale web-based study of adults with TTM (Woods et al., 2006), TTM in adults is associated with significant anxiety, depression, stress, social avoidance, and functional impairment. The functional impact of the symptoms can sometimes result in "derailing" from expected developmental trajectories to the point where even when the TTM is under much better control the consequences of having had TTM for decades sometimes remains. For example, approximately 75% of the participants involved in the Trichotillomania Impact Study reported that TTM interfered significantly with studying, and about 5% reported having dropped out of school directly as a result of TTM's effects on their lives (Woods et al., 2006). For patients whose lives have been so disrupted by TTM, it is imperative to pay clinical attention to matters of improving day-to-day functioning, such as re-establishing professional and personal contacts, developing greater confidence in their ability to cope with life's other challenges, determining what to do with the time now regained from engaging in hours of TTM-related behaviors and concealment of damage caused by pulling, mending fences with loved ones caught in TTM's crossfire, and building a life without TTM that is meaningful and sufficiently challenging. Patients who have been unemployed or underemployed for years because of TTM-related disability fear that the return to gainful employment will trigger recurrence of symptoms and are thus reluctant to take on these challenges, yet also fear that failing to do so will leave them with too much idle time than is likely to be healthy. It is important to carefully assess the challenges that face the TTM patient who is completing a successful course of CBT, since problems in re-integrating into their social roles can threaten the stability of the treatment gains by increasing stress. We encourage our patients at this stage of treatment to consider returning to or developing new hobbies (e.g., exercise regimen) that can help fill in the idle time and increase their sense of accomplishment and worth, both of which are often compromised by the effects of TTM. In our recent clinical studies of child and adolescent patients, we devoted the first eight weeks (eight sessions) to establishing the treatment regimen, and then devoted four more sessions over eight weeks to maintenance of gains; it was during this latter phase that issues about re-integration, lifestyle changes, etc. were emphasized, but in clinical practice this could be extended beyond the eight-week maintenance period in response to the degree of patient impairment and the need for clinical time devoted to devising and implementing a clinical plan for maintaining gains associated with CBT and improvement of functioning. We expect that continued functional impairment and avoidance is stressful, and hence a risk factor for the development of increased urges, pulling, and relapse. Thus, the importance of addressing functioning via problem solving cannot be underemphasized.

MAINTENANCE CASE EXAMPLE

We present here a case example to help summarize the material presented above. Rachel presented for CBT after having already tried several other treatment methods including SSRIs and hypnosis. Rachel's TTM symptoms primarily involved scalp pulling, included both unfocused pulling during sedentary activities and focused pulling in response to stress (e.g., "I need to go pull to calm myself down"), and avoidance of many social situations and opportunities to get involved in interpersonal and romantic relationships, which she typically eschewed because "nobody would understand the pulling."

Acute treatment progressed in accordance with the outline above: Rachel learned more about the specific patterns of pulling, which environmental and affective cues were associated with increasing urges to pull, and her tendency to catastrophize when she found herself engaging in unfocused pulling and the subsequent effects of this kind of thinking on her mood and pulling behavior later on ("now that I've started I might as well keep doing it"). This information led to the development of a comprehensive and tailored approach that incorporated self-monitoring of pulling and of playing with her hair (a precursor to unfocused pulling for Rachel), stimulus control methods such as hats, bandanas, and band-aids in situations that were high risk for unfocused pulling (e.g., reading, computer time), and development of several habit reversal techniques for use when urges were evident (e.g., fist clenching, playing with stuffed animal when experiencing urges to pull when home alone). Acute treatment progressed nicely – Rachel was highly motivated, interested in understanding the specifics of her TTM better, and figuring out how to stay one step ahead of her urges to pull. She was able to curtail her pulling behavior almost completely by the end of acute treatment, although she still had occasional urges to pull that were stronger when she was feeling especially emotional.

With the core techniques in place, the work during maintenance shifted to improving Rachel's general functioning and to encouraging her to confront personal challenges rather than avoiding them out of fear that doing so would exacerbate the TTM urges. Rachel was pleased with the progress she had made during acute treatment and was heavily invested in protecting her treatment gains; in the view of the therapist, this approach actually exposed Rachel to increased risk of relapse because her interpersonal and professional life had been substantially compromised by TTM, and avoiding opportunities to improve these areas of her life would likely be associated with more negative emotion, more free time, increased boredom, and hence more urges to pull. Below is a depiction of the discussion about these issues that was addressed in a maintenance session.

T: Nice to see you again – how are things?

P: Going pretty well, thanks.

T: Keeping up with the program thus far?

P: Yeah – the idea to put baskets together for every room with gloves, hats, and stuff to play with in them is really helping.

T: *Good – anything that makes it easier for you to implement the techniques before the urges arise is going to be in your best interests – why rely on your motivation at 11 pm to get up and go find gloves?*

P: *You're right – I'm leaving the baskets right where I need them, and then I don't have any excuses for not using them.*

T: *And the more you use them now, the weaker the urges will get.*

P: *It's interesting – I actually asked my Dad last week about his urges to smoke, which he hasn't done in about ten years, and he said the same thing: right after he quit he used to have to leave the dinner table right away and take a long walk because that was a time of strong urges to smoke so he needed to get away from all that. Now though he says he can sit at the table after dinner talking and he doesn't have any urges.*

T: *That's the idea – use the techniques until the urges truly dissipate, and then fade them if you want to later on.*

P: *Not sure I'll want to fade them, because they're easy to do and I don't want to take any unnecessary chances.*

T: *You're really invested in keeping this going – good for you!*

P: *I am – I've come a long way.*

T: *What have you noticed about the urges in the last few weeks?*

P: *Well I'm being pretty diligent in the high risk places so I don't find myself absent mindedly playing with my hair, which probably is why I'm having fewer urges in general.*

T: *And how about the urges associated with strong negative emotions?*

P: *Those I'm still getting, but I'm still being pretty good about not letting myself give in – using the habit reversal stuff instead. It's not easy and it never does feel quite the same way as pulling would, but when the urges go down I wind up feeling pretty proud of myself for riding it out.*

T: *All good – nice to hear.*

P: *I'm still thinking though about the stuff we talked about last time – finishing college, getting out more, that kind of stuff.*

T: *And?*

P: *Well it still seems really risky to me – I dropped out of school last time because of the pulling while I was trying to study, and I'm still not sure that I'm ready to handle relationships yet.*

T: *So you're worried that increasing the stress level by re-enrolling in school and trying to get yourself out there more socially would threaten the treatment gains?*

P: *(Hesitates) Yeah, I guess that's how I'm looking at it.*

T: Understandable – you worked really hard to get this under control, so who wouldn't want to protect that? It's perfectly natural.

P: I guess.

T: There's another side to it, though, isn't there? Changing those things in your life that you aren't happy with would indeed be stressful, but so would not changing them?

P: Sure – I'm not really happy working at the restaurant, and I think I can do better.

T: Better in what way?

P: You know, education-wise and financially.

T: And you see those two things as linked?

P: I think so – I'm not too many credits short of my B.A., and I'm not really in any position financially to do anything other than continue to work at the restaurant.

T: So you're thinking about down the road.

P: I am, but every time I do I remember what it was like to try to study with trich in full force and then I just put off thinking about it.

T: There's something you're not taking into consideration, though – you're not in the same position you used to be with respect to your knowledge of TTM and how to keep it at bay, are you?

P: I suppose not, but I expect that the urges will go up if I try to finish my degree.

T: Oh, I agree with you completely – you can probably bank on it. However, as we've talked about in here a lot, the presence of an urge does not necessarily dictate what your response must be, and that's what you've learned in CBT: you're vulnerable to urges more than most people, maybe because of neurobiology, but that doesn't necessarily paint you into a corner in terms of responses. Biology isn't destiny, after all – even the hard-core geneticists would agree to that.

P: True, but it will be work, expensive, and probably make it harder to maintain my gains.

T: Let's say we expand what you mean by your gains, however. Let's say we include not only trich symptoms specifically but the associated functional impairment, reticence to take on big challenges for fear of tipping the apple cart, and reluctance to live the life you've imagined.

If we broaden what we consider under the umbrella of TTM's effects on your life it seems like it's pretty important to expand our efforts to work on functioning better and doing what you want to do with your life – after all, if you don't ever pull again but don't accomplish your life's bigger goals, I'm not sure anyone would be satisfied with that as an outcome. Learning the techniques and getting it under control certainly was and still is an important target, which is why we emphasized it so much during the first part of the treatment, but if we simply stop here then I'm not sure that will be enough for you to feel that you're living a satisfying and enjoyable life. And if I'm right, and I think I am, that could lead to increased negative emotions to handle down the road, which in turn could feed back into increasing urges to pull, more pulling behavior, and thus imperil the very thing you're trying so hard to maintain.

P: It's going to be hard, though.

T: Sure it will, but it will also open other doors for you as well – you've said for a long time that you don't feel like you connect well with the folks you work with, yet you don't have a ton of other outlets socially.

P: I did start volunteering again at the church, mainly clerical stuff but sometimes other stuff.

T: That's great – it's more time out of your apartment when you're not working, an opportunity to meet people and be helpful, and maybe that too can lead to some other opportunities.

P: It's important to me, and I know that my Mom is happy that I'm doing that again.

T: Great to hear – a really good step.

P: I'm trying not to isolate myself so much now, although I'm still very reluctant to get close to people and to disclose what I've been through.

T: Understandable, and something that you'll be able to decide as you spend more time with people and feel them out for their ability to be accepting. Disclosure is probably a lot harder at a bus stop with complete strangers than it would be with people who you know well and with whom you have a lot in common.

P: (Laughs). Can you imagine – announcing that I had trich at the train station?

T: Well it's a lot more common than we used to think and you might be surprised, but I agree that it's reasonable to be discerning with who you decide to tell and who you don't. Have you disclosed your pulling to anyone?

P: Well my parents and my sisters know, and I'm sure some people used to suspect, but I've been really cautious with that.

T: Because you're afraid that people won't get it? That's what you told me when you first got here – do you still feel that way?

P: I do, I guess.

T: And I'm guessing that has something to do with being reluctant to go out with friends, pursue new relationships, and try to meet people?

P: Probably – if you meet people and get to know them well, at some point you're going to have to cross that bridge if you have TTM.

T: Maybe especially so when you're dating someone?

P: Right.

T: Again, though, let's expand the definition of trich's effects to include your ability to pursue relationships and find deep and lasting connections with other people. If that aspect of your life remains impaired for fear that disclosure will be stressful or out of concern that the stress of doing so will be stressful and lead to increase urges to pull, does that seem like a tradeoff you're willing to make in the long run?

P: No, not really – I want to be closer to other people and I want to meet someone special, but I also want to maintain the progress I've made on my trich.

T: And right now those things seem mutually exclusive to you?

P: I don't think I'd really thought it through quite so much until now, but yeah – it feels like taking those risks personally might threaten my progress with trich.

T: Only if we have a narrow definition of progress, right? If the only thing that matters is reducing hairpulling then you might be right – all stress should be avoided lest it disrupt the program's effectiveness. On the other hand, failing to push forward on these really important life goals is probably stressful as well, so I'm not sure that your premise is accurate.

P: Maybe not.

T: (Seizing an opportunity to match a metaphor to the interests and vocabulary of the patient in front of him): You're dilemma sort of reminds me of the Parable of the Talents, you know, from the Old Testament? If you're so concerned about losing your fortune that you go dig a hole and bury it in a field then you ensure that you won't lose it – on the other hand you won't gain much from having amassed it, nor will the people around you.

P: I see your point.

T: Well then maybe some of work we do going forward will involve making a specific plan and timeline for moving forward with the things you want to improve in your life.

P: That sounds good.

CONCLUSION

"The better you do the better you will do," is one of the summary statements that can be derived both from the empirical literature on disorders other than TTM and from our collective clinical experience with TTM. Accordingly, the clinical approaches to psychoeducation, treatment planning, and using CBT techniques that are described in detail above are recommended as strategies for helping patient not only make but also maintain clinically significant improvement, and should be discussed as such from the very beginning of acute treatment. We also emphasize early on that CBT for TTM is best thought of from a teaching perspective, in that patients will learn from their therapists specific strategies and ways to cope more effectively with urges to pull. By emphasizing the transfer of control and responsibility for treatment over the course of the therapy, we seek to empower the patient and help them "own" the progress that is made during CBT. It is especially important to do this since CBT is typically a short-term treatment that comes with the explicit expectation (at least when presented by us) that the patient's symptoms are not likely to be completely eradicated by the end of the acute phase, nor will the vulnerability to obsessions be expunged forever. The patient should be encouraged that their new-found knowledge of how to deal with their pulling behaviors and urges when they inevitably arise and improved ability to quickly recognize new obsessions and knowledge of what to do when confronted with new urges leave them in a better position to battle TTM successfully in the long run. Therapists should be sure to encourage the use of booster sessions in accordance with their patients' needs, and should generally leave the door open for contact in the future should the need arise.

TREATMENT: ADJUNCTIVE MODULES

Introduction to Part 3: Modules

In the preceding section we have provided a detailed account and clinical examples of how to present the rationale for and to implement the core techniques of CBT for TTM, which include awareness training, stimulus control, competing response training, and maintenance. In our view clinically this package constitutes the foundation upon which TTM treatment should be based, and the available research data attest to the efficacy and durability of this protocol. Nevertheless, the empirical data on TTM in adults suggest that relapse following treatment with CBT protocols containing these elements is not uncommon, and recently clinical researchers have begun to consider adjunctive or alternative approaches to the treatment of this chronic problem. From several recent reviews of this literature it appears that there may be need for affect management strategies to help with pulling behavior that is clearly serving some strong affective function (e.g., Linehan, 1993). From a clinical standpoint it is important to examine with the patient during the early stages of awareness training the degree to which intense emotions (e.g., depression, anger) are linked to urges to pull and pulling behavior. Accordingly, we have included in the manual several modules that we have found useful on a case-by-case basis to help modulate the effects of affect on pulling. These include relaxation training/stress management procedures for patients who report that their TTM is linked to anxiety, stress, and muscle tension, and cognitive restructuring for those whose irrational thinking contributes either directly or indirectly to pulling behavior.

We have also included in this section a module on motivational enhancement – although many of our TTM patients come to treatment ready and willing to "work the program," others are less intrinsically or extrinsically motivated to reduce pulling behavior. Moreover, even in patients who start treatment with enthusiasm, motivation can wane over time, and thus a module on motivational enhancement struck us as especially important to include with this manual. One of us (DFT) has developed a motivational program based on the work on Motivational Interviewing by Miller and Rollnick (2002) and tailored for use with adult OCD patients who initially refused CBT. An empirical study of that protocol indicated that compared to a control condition, the motivational enhancement program was successful in helping patients re-engage and enter treatment (Maltby & Tolin, 2005). We have tailored our discussion of motivational issues here to address the specific issues that often arise in TTM.

In addition to the modules on relaxation/stress management, cognitive restructuring, and motivational enhancement, we also decided to include two other modules in this section, one on group treatment and other supportive methods, and another on family-based approaches. There is now at least some study of the efficacy of group approaches for TTM in adults, and they may be thought to play an adjunctive role in treatment; one of the primary advantages of group approaches is that they by their very nature allow patients to recognize that they are not the only ones struggling with TTM and related problems. Group treatments can range from those that are designed specifically to teach the same CBT techniques we discuss here to those that are much more focused on providing support for participants; both will be discussed in turn. The development of web-based technologies that allow patients to access information about TTM and its treatment may also be a way to improve access to care – we discuss in that module the program called Stoppulling.com, which was developed for this purpose and now has empirical support for its efficacy (Mouton-Odum et al., 2006).

Family-based approaches certainly make logical sense for younger patients and although they have been advocated they have generally not been subjected to empirical testing; such approaches are imperative when the presenting patient is a toddler or pre-schooler or when negative family interactions about TTM and other matters predicts pulling behavior (Wright et al., 2003). Families of children and adolescents obviously play a critical role in the delivery of even the core modules, and in this section on family factors we will expand on how we try to work with families of children and adolescents across the developmental spectrum; for those who are focusing on treatment of children and adolescents we suggest reading the family section even before delivering the core modules, lest family factors arise in treatment that require specific clinical attention.

We encourage those who have purchased the manual to review the material contained in these as-needed modules to determine whether and how they might be incorporated into the clinical management of clinical patients with TTM that you encounter in clinical practice. For those clinicians who work primarily with children and adolescents, the chapter on family-based approaches might be useful background reading in anticipation of difficulties and clinical decisions to be made in response to emergent family issues.

CHAPTER 11

I'M NOT SURE IF I'M READY:

Motivational Enhancement

By now, the reader should have a sense that CBT is a potentially useful way of addressing the complex problems of TTM. The reader may also surmise, quite correctly, that successful implementation of CBT is no easy task. Perhaps the most important factor that distinguishes CBT from more traditional forms of psychotherapy is the fact that it is active and effortful, rather than passive. Whereas traditional psychotherapy is based primarily on conversations between therapist and patient, CBT adds a number of active exercises, not all of which are pleasant, that the patient must practice regularly.

This level of effort on the patient's part requires that the patient be at least reasonably motivated to change, and remain so throughout the treatment. Most therapists (ourselves included) can easily think of several examples in which a patient's low or fluctuating motivation presented an obstacle to successful implementation of treatment strategies. Some illustrative case examples are presented below.

Carl, a 13-year-old boy, was brought to treatment by his mother. His mother seemed very much at the end of her rope, and she made repeated statements such as, "I can't stand to see him doing this to himself." Carl presented with marked alopecia; he had two large bald patches on his scalp, and he had no eyebrows or eyelashes. Surprisingly, however, Carl seemed relatively unfazed by the problem. When the therapist asked Carl whether he thought he had a hair-pulling problem, he replied, "Not really. Sure, I pull my hair, but it's really no big deal."

The therapist then asked Carl whether he thought he had a significant amount of hair loss, enough that other children could notice it. The therapist was astonished to hear Carl say, "I don't really think other kids notice it that much. No one's ever mentioned it to me." Later in the session, the therapist learned the Carl had very little social contact with peers. He did not talk to classmates at school, and ate his lunch alone at the cafeteria. It seemed, therefore, that Carl's lack of social feedback about his appearance may have been a byproduct of his lack of social contact in general. The therapist moved forward, suggesting interventions such as competing response training and stimulus control. Although Carl attended therapy sessions regularly, he rarely followed through with homework assignments. At the end of his treatment, there was little improvement in his hair pulling or alopecia.

Other patients may initially present as highly motivated to change. However, their motivation appears to wane as assignments become more challenging. Sarah, a 26-year-old woman, was such a patient. At the initial session, Sarah appeared highly distressed by her hair pulling and the resulting loss of hair on her eyebrows. She said, "I'll try just about anything if it will help me stop pulling." The therapist perceived this and related statements as a "green light" to move forward with interventions. In the early sessions, Sarah seemed like the perfect patient. She completed her self-monitoring homework diligently, and was eager to participate in discussions with the therapist about her hair pulling and its antecedents and consequences. Sarah also seemed to enjoy learning relaxation exercises (see Chapter 12), and reported practicing these exercises every day. However, when the therapist began competing response training, Sarah became much less cooperative with treatment. After one week of homework assignments, Sarah complained that the intervention seemed too difficult and time-consuming. She began to make statements she had not made before, such as, "I'm not sure my hair pulling is so bad that I really need to do all of this." She also stated, "It's not fair that I have to do all this work just because I pull my hair."

Such instances of flagging or absent motivation to change are common in the treatment of TTM. In fact, our experience has been that a certain degree of ambivalence is the rule, rather than the exception. Patients alternatively, or perhaps even simultaneously, want to change their behavior, and do not want to change. Certainly there is ample reason for TTM patients to be ambivalent about change, given the amount of negative and/or positive reinforcement that accompanies pulling. Furthermore, overcoming these disorders is often hard work, and it is difficult for many people to sustain a consistently high degree of motivation.

Miller and Rollnick (2002) addressed this problem with the development of Motivational Interviewing (MI). Although MI was originally developed in the context of alcohol and substance abuse treatment, many of its principles seem to fit TTM treatment quite well. MI is best conceptualized not as a specific treatment or technique, but rather as a basic way of understanding patients' ambivalence and overcoming resistance to change. Thus, a "flavor" of MI is present throughout all of treatment, often from the initial session.

The model of MI is based on the premise that motivation to change is not a stable personality trait. Rather, it is a state of readiness that may fluctuate over time. Prochaska and DiClemente (1982) identified six "stages of change," shown in Table 11.1. Different therapist approaches are needed for clients in different stages, as noted in the Table. Miller and Rollnick suggest that patients may cycle back and forth between these stages, sometimes several times, before permanent change is achieved. Furthermore, a person may be motivated to change one behavior but not another, to adhere to a certain treatment but not another, or to see one therapist but not another.

Another key assumption of MI is that responsibility for motivation lies with the therapist, not with the patient. This is radically different from traditional clinical thinking, in which it is common for a therapist to say, "This patient's just not motivated." MI therapists, on the other hand, would be more likely to say, "What can I do to help this patient decide to change their behavior?"

This, of course, is the million-dollar question. How can the therapist, faced with an ambivalent or "unmotivated" patient, help that patient to reach the conclusion that he/she needs to change his/her behavior? The MI model suggests that ambivalent patients usually cannot be persuaded by direct or aggressive confrontation; instead, such interventions tend to lead to counter-arguments. Patients are most likely to decide to change *when they themselves make the argument for*

Table 11.1. Stages of Change and Associated Therapist Tasks

Stage of Change	Therapist's Motivational Tasks
Precontemplation	The patient needs awareness, information, and feedback about TTM. Raise doubt—increase the patient's perception of risks and problems with hair pulling.
Contemplation	The patient needs to talk about the possibility of working on hair pulling, and is likely to waver back and forth. The therapist's task is to tip the balance in favor of change by evoking reasons to stop pulling, and risks of not stopping.
Determination	The patient has made a decision to try to stop pulling. This is a "window of opportunity" for the therapist to help the patient find a strategy that is acceptable, accessible, appropriate, and effective. Help the patient to determine the best course of action to take.
Action	Help the patient to take steps to stop pulling.
Maintenance	Help the patient to identify and use strategies to prevent relapse.
Relapse	Help the patient to renew the process of contemplation, determination, and action, without becoming stuck or demoralized because of relapse. Help the patient to resume maintenance efforts.

Adapted from Miller, W., & Rollnick, S. (2002). *Motivational interviewing: Preparing people for change* (2nd ed.). New York: Guilford. Get permission *change*. That is, the therapist's job is not to persuade the patient to change, or provide them with a list of reasons why they should change. Rather, the MI therapist works to elicit and reinforce self-motivational statements from the patient. Miller and Rollnick (2002) list four categories of self-motivational statements: Problem recognition (e.g., a statement that one has a problem), expression of concern (e.g., a statement that the problem is serious, or that help is needed), intention to change (e.g., a statement that one has decided to do something about the problem), and optimism (e.g., a statement that it is possible to change the problem, and that one is capable of doing it). Again, however, it is emphasized that these statements are most helpful if they come from the patient, not from the therapist.

THE PRINCIPLES OF MOTIVATIONAL INTERVIEWING

The general principles of MI are summarized in Table 11.2. The first (and perhaps most important) therapeutic strategy is to express empathy for the patient's ambivalence. One of the most straightforward ways to do this is to use the Rogerian strategy of reflective listening. Reflective listening may include some or all of the following components:

Table 11.2. The Principles of Motivational Interviewing

Principle	Corollaries
Express empathy	Acceptance facilitates change. Skillful listening is fundamental. Ambivalence is normal.
Develop discrepancy	Awareness of the consequences of hair pulling is important. A discrepancy between hair pulling and important goals will motivate change. The patient should present the arguments for stopping hair pulling.
Avoid argumentation	Arguments are counterproductive. Defending breeds defensiveness. Resistance is a signal to change strategies. Labeling is unnecessary.
Roll with resistance	Momentum can be used to good advantage. Perceptions can be shifted. New perspectives are invited but not imposed. The patient is a valuable resource in finding solutions to problems.
Support self-efficacy	Belief in the possibility of reducing hair pulling is an important motivator. The patient is responsible for choosing their method of stopping hair pulling, and carrying out the plan. There is hope in the range of alternative approaches available.

Adapted from Miller, W., & Rollnick, S. (2002). *Motivational interviewing: Preparing people for change* (2nd ed.). New York: Guilford. Get permission

- Open-ended questions about the rewarding aspects of the problem behavior.
  - "What are some good things about hair pulling?"
  - "What do you like and dislike about pulling?"
- Statements, rather than questions, about what you think the patient means.
  - "Hair pulling doesn't seem to be a very big deal to you right now."
  - "The amount of work in involved in overcoming hair pulling doesn't really seem worth it to you."
- Reflecting what the patient seems to be feeling.
  - "You look frustrated right now."
  - "You're feeling pretty overwhelmed."
- Selectively emphasizing certain aspects of what was said, to move the patient toward more self-motivational statements.
  - "I hear you saying that the other kids having mentioned that they notice your bald spots. You also mentioned that they don't say much at all to you, because you don't hang out with other kids very much at school. Tell me more about how the other kids treat you."
  - "You've said that you like the way pulling makes you feel, but you don't like the way it makes you look. Can you tell me more about what it is about the way you look that bothers you?"
- Using compliments and statements of appreciation and understanding.
  - "This has been a very difficult problem for you to even talk about, and I think you're being very brave by talking to me today."
  - "You're right, these exercises really are difficult and they take a lot of time. I appreciate the fact that you've been willing to work so hard."
- Making summary statements to link together material that has been discussed, particularly self-motivational statements.
  - "So there are some good things and some bad things about hair pulling. On the one hand, hair pulling feels pretty good to you, and so far, no one has told you that they notice your bald spots. On the other hand, you've also mentioned that you don't hang out with other kids is much as you'd like to, and you suspect that this might be because they do notice your bald spots and so they treat you differently."
  - "You've raised some very important points about the work we're doing. It's pretty difficult, and sometimes it takes up time that you could be using to do something else. You've also mentioned, though, that hair pulling is even more time-consuming than these exercises, and that it's really impacting how you feel about yourself."

Another principle of MI is to develop discrepancy between the patient's problem behavior and their life goals. The goal of this intervention is to help the patient recognize the consequences of their behavior. The patient becomes more strongly motivated to change when they understand that the problem behavior is fundamentally inconsistent with other things that are important to them. Strategies for developing discrepancy include:

- Using summary statements to summarize ambivalence.
  - "You've told me that you would like to have more friends. How does your hair pulling fit with that goal?"
  - "On one hand, you like your free time and don't want to be bothered with a bunch of time-consuming exercises. On the other hand, getting control of this hair pulling problem also seems to be important for you."
- Eliciting self-motivational statements. Some ways to elicit self-motivational statements include:
  - Evocative questions: "What leads you to think that that hair pulling has become a problem?" "In what ways does your hair pulling concern you?" "What makes you think that you might need to make a change here?" "What makes you think that if you did decide to stop pulling, you could do it?"
  - Elaboration: "You mentioned that your hair pulling bugs you sometimes. Tell me more about that." "What did you mean when you said that it's important to you to stop pulling?"
  - Using extremes: "What do you suppose are the worst things that can happen if you keep pulling?"
  - Looking back: "What was your life like before you started pulling hair? How does it compare to your life now?"
  - Looking forward: "How would you like things to turn out for you?"
  - Exploring goals: "What things are really important to you? Where does pulling hair rank among these things? How does pulling move you toward or away from those other goals?"

Miller and Rollnick (2002) caution that the therapist should avoid argumentation. According to the MI model, arguments between the therapist and patient usually result in the patient becoming more, not less, resistant to change. The more strongly the therapist makes the case for change, the more the patient tends to dig in his/her heels. Some conversational styles to avoid include:

- Ordering, directing, or commanding
- Warning or threatening
- Giving advice, making suggestions, or providing solutions
- Persuading with logic, arguing, or lecturing
- Moralizing, preaching, or telling patients what they "should" do
- Criticizing, blaming, or labeling
- Interpreting or analyzing
- Asking rapid-fire questions
- Reminding the patient how serious his/her problem is
- Insisting on talking about the problem behavior when the patient has other concerns he/she wants to discuss

An important goal of MI is to roll with resistance. Often, even a well-meaning therapist may inadvertently elicit or strengthen resistance. In MI, patient resistance is considered to be directly related to the therapist's behaviors; therefore, therapists can decrease (or increase) resistance by changing their style. When the patient exhibits resistance, this should serve as a signal that the therapist is using strategies that are not appropriate for the patient's stage of change. Miller and Rollnick (2002) identify four categories of patient resistance behavior: arguing (contesting the therapist's accuracy, expertise, or integrity), interrupting (breaking in and interrupting in a defensive manner), denying (expressing an unwillingness to recognize problems, cooperate, accept responsibility, or take advice), and ignoring (showing evidence of ignoring or not following the therapist). Strategies for handling resistance include:

- Simple reflection: "Your hair pulling doesn't seem like a big deal to you."
- Amplified reflection, in the hope of getting the patient to back off a bit from their initial resistance: "Your hair pulling seems like a good thing to you."
- Double-sided reflection, in which the resistance statement is reflected and paired with a self-motivational statement mentioned earlier: "These exercises seem really difficult, and, as you mentioned to me before, overcoming hair pulling is a high priority for you."
- Shifting focus, when resistance is strong and does not seem that further discussion will be fruitful: "Let's switch gears for a bit. Can you tell me how school is going for you?"
- Agreement with a twist, in which an initial agreement is paired with a slight change of direction: "You're absolutely right that these exercises are hard. Sometimes, it takes hard work to overcome a difficult problem."
- Emphasizing personal choice and control: "Ultimately, the decision about whether to work on your hair pulling is yours. I can provide you with some guidance, but I can't tell you what you should or should not do."
- Reframing, or offering a new meaning or interpretation of the patient's observations: "You've mentioned that other kids haven't said anything to you about your bald spots. But as you've been telling me more about how things go for you at school, I'm hearing that the other kids don't talk much to you at all, and you end up feeling lonely."

The final principle of MI is supporting the patient's self-efficacy to change. Because the patient's stage of change is likely to fluctuate over time, there is a window of opportunity during which the therapist can help the patient to move toward action. Signs that the patient may be ready to make this move include:

- Decreased resistance (patient stops arguing or objecting).
- Decreased questions about the problem (patient seems to have enough information).
- Resolve (patient appears to have reached a resolution to change, and may seem more relaxed or peaceful).

- Self-motivational statements (patient makes direct self-motivational statements reflecting problem recognition, concern, openness to change, or optimism about their ability to change).
- Increased questions about change (patient asks what he/she can do about the problem, or how people stop pulling once they have decided to).
- Envisioning (patient talks about how life might be after they stop pulling).
- Experimenting (patient has begun experimenting with change strategies).

Miller and Rollnick (2002) caution that this is a delicate phase in the patient's transition to action. The main hazard at this point is underestimating the patient's degree of ambivalence. Most decision is to change our may gradually, not all at once, and the therapist should take care not to confuse the decision-making process with an actual decision. The therapist must discern, therefore, whether the patient is thinking out loud about their options, or whether he/she has actually made up his/her mind. Once it is clear that the patient has committed to change his/her behavior, the role of the therapist is to channel this motivation into a workable plan for change. The patient's freedom of choice should be reiterated throughout this process; for example, the therapist might discuss the pros and cons of taking medications versus receiving CBT, and ask the patient what he/she wants to do. Once an initial treatment plan has been developed, the patient's motivation may be strengthened further by setting both short- and long-term goals.

The therapist may provide the patient with a change plan worksheet, in which the patient responds to items such as:

- The most important reasons why I want to stop pulling are . . .
- My main goals for myself, in stopping pulling, are . . .
- I plan to do these things in order to reach my goals:
- The first steps that I plan to take to stop pulling are . . .
- Other people could help me to stop pulling in these ways:
- I hope that my plan will have these positive results:

CHAPTER 12

CALMING DOWN:

Module 2: Relaxation and Other Stress-Management Strategies

Relaxation exercises have a long history in medicine and mental health treatment (Jacobson, 1929). Indeed, entire treatments for anxiety disorders have been based around variants of muscle relaxation (e.g., Haugen, Dixon, & Dickel, 1963). Within the anxiety disorders, the rationale for relaxation exercises is based on the tripartite model of anxiety (e.g., Lang, 1979), in which anxious physiology, cognition, and behavior are thought to mutually influence one another in a positive or negative direction. In the positive direction, symptoms of sympathetic nervous system arousal (often termed the "fight or flight" response) lead to an increase in worried thoughts and escape or avoidance behavior. In the negative direction, reductions in physiological arousal are presumed to lead to reductions in anxious thoughts and behaviors.

Countless forms of relaxation training have been developed, and in general, there seem to be few differences in efficacy among these different interventions. One of the more common variants of relaxation training is progressive muscle relaxation (PMR). PMR involves focusing sequentially on different parts of the body, tensing and then relaxing the muscles. Muscles are tensed before they are relaxed, in order to increase the patient's awareness of muscle tension in various parts of the body. Theoretically, increased awareness of muscle tension results in the patient's increased ability to detect and remedy such tension. The muscle tension may also serve to amplify the sensation of relaxation due to contrast effects, thus allowing the patient to understand more clearly what it feels like to relax a specific part of their body.

In an early study, progressive muscle relaxation was found to reduce feelings of tension among anxious college students. Participants who tensed, and then relaxed, their muscles, showed a somewhat better response than did patients who were only asked to relax their muscles (Borkovec, Grayson, & Cooper, 1978). Subsequent studies have demonstrated the efficacy of relaxation training for health concerns such as hypertension (Agras, Southam, & Taylor, 1983; Brauer, Horlick, Nelson, Farquhar, & Agras, 1979), chronic pain (Turner, 1982), headaches (Blanchard et al., 1982), and irritable bowel syndrome (Keefer & Blanchard, 2001); as well as anxiety-related problems such as dental anxiety (M. P. Miller, Murphy, & Miller, 1978), agoraphobia (Michelson, Mavissakalian, & Marchione, 1985), and generalized anxiety disorder (Borkovec & Costello, 1993). We note, however, that relaxation is rarely used as a stand-alone treatment for anxiety disorders. In fact, other forms of cognitive-behavioral therapy have been found to be superior to relaxation training alone (Borkovec & Costello, 1993; Clark et al., 1994; Greist et al., 2002), and in some cases (e.g., the treatment of panic disorder) the addition of relaxation training to other treatment components may even detract from treatment efficacy (Murphy, Michelson, Marchione, Marchione, & Testa, 1998; Schmidt et al., 2000).

The specific efficacy of relaxation training for TTM has not been established. We suspect that it is unlikely that many patients will find relaxation alone to be an effective treatment, and we generally consider other interventions such as self-monitoring, awareness training, competing response training and stimulus control to represent the "core" elements of TTM/BFRB treatment. However, it is likely that some patients will find that reducing their degree of physiological arousal will result in reduced urges to pull. Specifically, those patients for whom subjective anxiety and/or physiological tension serve as a trigger for pulling (see Chapter 2) may benefit from alternative strategies to reduce their discomfort. Furthermore, we have encountered some patients for whom abbreviated relaxation strategies can be used successfully as a competing response in habit reversal training.

We incorporated PMR in our protocol for children and adolescents with TTM. Although we did not measure the specific efficacy of PMR compared to the other components, we did ask patients to monitor their utilization of the different techniques learned in therapy, as well as the perceived usefulness of each compo-nent. Surprisingly, we found that most patients reported that they did not use PMR regularly, and rated PMR as less helpful than other components such as self-monitoring, competing response training, and stimulus control (Tolin et al., 2002). Using the same methodology with adults receiving group therapy for TTM, similar results were obtained: patients did not use the PMR exercises frequently, and reported finding them significantly less helpful than the "core" techniques (Brady et al., 2005). This finding adds to our belief that relaxation is not a critical component of CBT for most patients with TTM. However, we noted that a few patients, specifically those with pronounced anxiety symptoms, made greater use of relaxation and rated it as more helpful. Thus, we suspect that some patients may benefit from the addition of PMR to their treatment regimen. With the possible exception of patients with panic disorder, there is little reason to believe that relaxation training will be harmful, other than the fact that it may take time away from more efficacious treatment components.

The decision of whether to add relaxation training, then, is based in part on differential diagnosis (see Chapter 3), as well as the functional analysis of the pulling behavior (see Chapter 4). Patients who meet criteria for a comorbid anxiety disorder (although perhaps not panic disorder) may benefit from the general tension-reducing effects of relaxation training. Patients whose antecedents to pulling include strong feelings of anxiety, nervousness, or tension, or who report that pulling leads to reduced feelings of anxiety, may also be candidates for relaxation training. Some patients also request that they be thought ways to relax, and, in the absence of any contraindications, relaxation training may be added. We note again, however, that at best, relaxation training should be considered an adjunct to the more active forms of TTM treatment such as awareness training, self-monitoring, competing response training, and stimulus control.

An interesting variation on traditional relaxation training is the use of Eastern meditation strategies such as mindfulness meditation. Mindfulness meditation, and other interventions based on this principle, differs from traditional relaxation in that the goal is not necessarily to bring one's level of physiological arousal directly under conscious control. Instead, one aim of mindfulness meditation is to undermine the individual's attempts to try to control their internal experience, and instead to learn to observe it objectively. In this sense, the process of mindfulness meditation might be thought of as the "opposite" of traditional relaxation, even though the observable effects might be quite similar. Hayes et al. (1999) use metaphors to explain this principle, such as observing one's thoughts and feelings as one would observe leaves floating down the stream. The patient is encouraged to refrain from "jumping into the stream" and trying to alter the course of the leaves. Mindfulness-based approaches have been used as an intervention for anxiety (J. J. Miller, Fletcher, & Kabat-Zinn, 1995), depression (Teasdale et al., 2000), chronic pain (Kabat-Zinn, Lipworth, & Burney, 1985), and borderline personality disorder (Linehan, 1993). Of particular interest for TTM is the emerging use of mindfulness in the treatment of OCD (Hannan & Tolin, 2005) and addictions (Marlatt, 1994), each of which bears some functional or symptomatic similarity to TTM. In such applications, patients are thought to use mindfulness and acceptance, rather than direct struggle, to deal with behavioral urges. For example, a patient might be instructed to notice the urge without acting on it, rather than engage in counterproductive strategies (such as pulling) to reduce the urge directly. A preliminary controlled trial suggests that mindfulness and acceptance may hold promise for TTM (Woods, Wetterneck, & Flessner, 2006). In this study, 25 adult patients with TTM were randomly assigned to wait list or to a combination of competing response training and acceptance and commitment therapy (ACT), in which patients were taught to accept, rather than combat, their urges to pull. They were also taught to regard their pulling-related cognitions (e.g., "If I do not pull, I will go crazy") as mental noise, rather than as literal truths. Results indicated that 66% of treated patients, vs. 8% of untreated patients, met criteria for clinically significant change. Furthermore, treated patients showed a 58% reduction in reported number of hairs pulled, compared to a 28% increase in the untreated group. Of course, the fact that treated patients received a combination of interventions makes it impossible to ascertain whether ACT contributed meaningfully to outcome, and when asked about the helpfulness of each component of the intervention, patients rated competing response techniques as most helpful. Thus, although acceptance and mindfulness strategies may be promising components of treatment, they cannot yet be considered substitutes for other interventions such as CRT.

TRANSCRIPT OF RELAXATION SESSION

Nora is a 56-year-old woman who is in treatment for TTM. She and her therapist have been using interventions such as awareness training, self-monitoring, stimulus control, and habit reversal. Nora has had moderate success with these interventions; however, she reported that she feels nervous and tense all the time, and that she is substantially more likely to pull hair when she feels this way. Therefore, the therapist decided to introduce relaxation training as an adjunct to the other treatment interventions. In this session, the therapist will use two common variants of relaxation training: progressive muscle relaxation and breathing retraining.

T: Nora, you've told me that you had some success stopping yourself from pulling. That's terrific. However, you've also told me that it feels like you're still having constant problems with anxiety and tension, and that these feelings tend to lead to pulling. Do I have that right?

N: That's right. It's really frustrating. I feel like I'm doing so well, but then the anxiety starts to come over me and it feels like all I can do to feel better is pull.

T: That happens sometimes. You are doing well, but these uncomfortable feelings that you experience are making it hard for you. What I'd like to do is teach you some ways to help get a better sense of control over your anxiety. I can promise that I can make your anxiety go away completely. But I think that with practice, you can teach yourself to feel a bit calmer, and maybe that will help you to feel stronger in the face of these urges.

N: I think that would really help.

T: Perhaps a first step in controlling anxiety is understanding it a little better. Often, we think of anxiety as being this overwhelming mess that comes on us all of a sudden, and we don't know where it's from what it's about. But it might be helpful to break into pieces and understand what each piece is and how they interact with each other. We can think of anxiety as consisting of three components: feelings, thoughts, and actions. Each of these parts of anxiety is separate, but they influence each other. For example, you were describing how you were feeling this morning, and how the anxiety seemed to come out of nowhere.

N: Yeah, it felt like I was just sitting there, minding my own business, and all of a sudden I was anxious.

T: Let's talk about the different feelings you were having. What did it feel like to be anxious? For example, what emotions or physical sensations were you having?

N: Well, my neck muscles felt kind of tense and achy. And my palms felt clammy and wet. Oh, and it felt like my heart was pounding too.

T: OK, so tense muscles, clammy palms, and pounding heart are the sensations you get when you're anxious. What was going through your mind?

N: I was sitting there thinking about all the things I had to do today. Like I had to come here for my appointment, and in one of the late. And I also knew that I had to go grocery shopping and get dinner ready.

T: Was there something anxious or worried about these thoughts?

N: I guess I was thinking that maybe I wasn't going to have enough time to do all those things today. And that I was thinking that if I didn't get dinner ready on time, my husband would ask me what I was doing all day, and we'd probably have an argument.

T: So here's another part of your anxiety: worrying that you're not going to get everything done, and worrying about what's going to happen. This is the thinking part of your anxiety. And when you were feeling anxious, what kind of actions did you do?

N: I was drumming my fingers on the tabletop. Then I got up and kind of paced around the kitchen for a while. I went over and worked on my grocery-shopping list, but then put it down because I was feeling anxious and paced some more.

T: These are anxious actions. So we see that you had some anxious feelings, some anxious thoughts, and some anxious actions. And can you see how these different things influence each other? For example, when you paced around the kitchen, did that help you to stop worrying, or did it make your muscles less tense?

N: No. In fact, it did the opposite. It made me more anxious and tense.

T: So when you experience one part of that "anxiety triangle," the other parts tend to follow. It's can go the other way, too: if you can reduce one part of your anxiety, you may notice that the other parts also tend to come down. That's the purpose of the exercise I want to show you today. I'm going to show you a new, non-anxious action, that I think will lead you to feel less anxious, and maybe think less anxious as well. (Taking out a tape recorder) I'm going to make a tape of us going through this exercise, so you can listen to it and try it at home. To start, let's both sit comfortably, with both feet on the floor, and our hands either in our laps or on the arms of the chair. I'm going to loosen my necktie, so I don't feel constricted. If you have anything constricting you or pinching you, you may want to loosen it. This exercise probably works best if we close our eyes. Let's take a moment and sit here, with our eyes closed, and just get used to it. (Pause) Good. This exercise is called progressive muscle relaxation. The word "progressive" means that we're going to go through the different parts of our body and relax them, one by one. Before we relax them, though, we're going to tighten them up so they feel tense. We're going to do this for a couple of reasons. First, tensing the muscle makes you more aware of it, so you know where that muscle is and what it feels like. Second, when we tense up the muscle, it's easier to feel the muscle relaxing later. This will make it easier for you to relax the muscle on your own, because you'll remember that sensations better. Do you have any questions about that?

N: No, I think I get it.

T: OK. So let's start with one part of our body. We're going to tense it, and then, when I tell you to, we're going to relax it. When we relax it, we're going to try to do that all at once, like we're throwing the tension out of the muscle. I'm going to do it right along with you. Let's start with the right hand. We can tense these muscles by making a fist. So make a fist now with your right hand. (Nora does so) Good. Feel all those muscles in your hand: the fingers, the palm, everything. Notice what all that tension feels like. Hold it. (Waits 10 seconds) Now, when I say, we're going to relax that hand all at once. Ready? Relax. Feel all the tension leaving your hand, and the muscles get nice and loose and relaxed. Notice how different that feels. It feels a lot better this way. You can let your hand relaxed some more, let the fingers get floppy, and feel all that tension leaving your muscles. (Waits 20 seconds) Very good. Now let's go on to another part of the body, and will do the same thing.

The therapist then followed the same procedure for other parts of the body, tensing, then relaxing the muscle. Although the order is not particularly important, a common progression for adults might be:

- Right hand
- Left hand
- Both forearms (tensed by bending the wrists backward)
- Both biceps
- Neck and shoulders (tensed by raising the shoulders upwards, as if to put the shoulders into the ears)

- Face (tensed by wrinkling the nose, furrowing the brow, and pursing the lips)
- Chest (tensed by drawing the shoulders forward and inward)
- Stomach
- Buttocks
- Thighs
- Calves (tensed by pressing the toes into the floor and raising the heels off the floor)
- Feet (tensed by making fists with one's feet)

Younger children may have difficulty maintaining attention to this exercise if it is lengthy. Therefore, we often use an abbreviated relaxation protocol such as:

- Hands and arms
- Shoulders, neck, and face
- Chest and stomach
- Legs and feet

T: Very good. Now your whole body is feeling nice and relaxed. Let's keep our eyes closed for a little while longer, and pay attention to our breathing. Sometimes people think that the most relaxing way to breathe is to take big, deep breaths. Actually, that way of breathing sometimes makes people feel even more anxious and tense. The trick is not to take giant breaths, but rather to breathe in a slow, controlled manner. One way that we can do this is to count while we breathe. I'd like you to try breathing in through your nose and out through your mouth, while I count. I'm going to count to four while you breathe in, and I'm going to count to six while you breathe out. Ready? Breathe in through your nose. (Counting at a rate of approximately one per second) 1, 2, 3, 4. Now breathe out through your mouth. 1, 2, 3, 4, 5, 6. In through your nose. 1, 2, 3, 4. And out through your mouth. 1, 2, 3, 4, 5, 6. That's good. Keep breathing like that, counting to yourself. When you feel ready, you don't have to change your breathing or stop feeling relaxed; you can just open your eyes and look at me.

After the initial relaxation training session, the therapist gave Nora the tape of the exercise, with instructions to practice relaxing twice per day while listening to the tape. The therapist added that once Nora got the hang of the exercise, the tape would be optional. However, it was emphasized that learning to relax was a bit like learning to drive, swim, or ride a bicycle—it is a complex skill that requires a good deal of practice. The therapist also cautioned Nora not to do the relaxation exercises only when she was feeling anxious, as this might prove too difficult. Rather, she was encouraged to find some time each day when she could be alone and uninterrupted, and practice at those times, even if she was feeling relatively calm already. In subsequent sessions, the therapist instructed Nora to try relaxing when she was feeling anxious, tense, or stressed. Nora also found that as she became more skilled at relaxing, she could shorten the procedure significantly with a brief tension and relaxation of a few key muscles (e.g., her neck and shoulders).

Occasionally, very anxious patients will worry that they are not "doing it right." They may forget the order of muscles to tense and relax, they may not be able to sustain exhalation for six seconds, and so forth. This type of worrying defeats the aims of relaxation training by creating one more thing for the patient to be anxious about. We often find it helpful to remind patients that the goal of relaxation training is not to do a perfect job, and it doesn't really matter whether they follow our instructions to the letter. What seems to be important is that patients understand the general principle of tension and relaxation, as well as slow, controlled breathing, and that they practice these regularly.

PROBLEM SOLVING AND TIME MANAGEMENT STRATEGIES

For some patients, effective stress management is less about learning to relax than about learning how to handle real-life situations effectively and efficiently. Knowing that a patient is anxious or tense, therefore, does not automatically mean that relaxation training will be necessary or even useful. At the risk of repeating ourselves, we reiterate that the selection of specific interventions must be based on a clear understanding of the patient's target symptoms, as well as their antecedents and consequences. Obtaining this level of understanding often requires several detailed discussions with the patient about his/her life, the stressors they face, and how they manage those stressors.

Jeff, an 18-year-old young man, reported chronic feelings of anxiety and worry. As the therapist got to know him a bit better, he learned that Jeff, who was in his senior year of high school, was planning to go to college but had not yet decided where to go. He was fortunate enough to have been accepted to a rather prestigious school; however, it was over a thousand miles away from home, and he was nervous about being so far away from his family. He had also been accepted to a State university that was approximately 20 miles from home. He reported feeling "stuck" and not knowing what to do.

Lisa, a 33-year-old divorced woman, identified herself as a "supermom" during the initial evaluation session. She had two children, both under the age of 5. She was working full time as an accountant, and her children were in day care. She tended to fall behind schedule at work because she spent an inordinate amount of time talking to friends and family members on the telephone. As a result, she had to remain at work late in order to finish her tasks. She would then rush home to pick up her children, and, after making them a quick dinner, would fall exhausted on the couch. She reported feeling fatigued all the time, and was finding it progressively harder to concentrate. She found that her busy schedule left her little time to exercise, socialize, or do her homework assignments.

In our opinion, patients such as these are not necessarily best served by learning relaxation exercises. Although such exercises might be helpful adjuncts, they would not address the core problems of problem-solving difficulties and poor time management. Specific training in these areas, therefore, may prove more effective ways to help these patients manage their stress levels.

Effective problem solving (where Jeff has become "stuck") consists of five operations. They do not necessarily occur in a fixed order, and people may move back and forth among these operations before reaching a satisfactory conclusion. For a more thorough review, the reader is referred to D'Zurilla and Nezu (1999).

- General orientation: The individual recognizes that a problem exists, and that it is potentially solvable. The individual stops their action, and thinks about the problem. In Jeff's case, the therapist taught him to say to himself, "Stop and think" when he noticed himself worrying about his decision.
- Problem definition and formulation: The individual identifies the problem as clearly as possible. Jeff's therapist helped him to recognize that he had two conflicting goals: on one hand, he wanted to attend the prestigious university; on the other hand, he wanted to remain closer to home.
- Generation of alternatives: The individual "brainstorms" possible solutions to the problem. During this operation, the aim is to generate as many alternatives as possible, even if they seem silly. For example, Jeff was able to identify each college as an alternative. He also entertained the possibility of taking a year off before going to college, and looking for a prestigious school in his area.
- Decision making: The individual weighs the pros and cons of each alternative. Factors to consider include the likely outcomes of each alternative, as well as the feasibility of alternatives. Jeff ruled out looking for a new college because he did not want to delay his planned career path for an extra year. He decided that it would be in his best interest to go to the university closer to home.
- Verification: Ideally, the individual takes the planned course of action, notes the outcome, and determines whether this was indeed the right choice. In Jeff's case, he was unable to determine objectively the "correctness" of his college choice right away. He was, however, able to notice that, having made the decision, he felt a sense of relief. This served as a signal to him that he had made a good choice, and did not need to continue problem solving.

Patients such as Lisa may benefit from time management training. Although one might think, given her career as an accountant, that Lisa would be highly efficient in all of her daily activities, in fact she appeared to use her time at work inefficiently at work. This inefficiency then spilled over into her life outside of work, which left her feeling exhasusted (and perhaps even less efficient at work the following day). There are several self-help references on the topic of time management, which many patients find useful (e.g., Lakein, 1973; Wong, 1994).

Although specific methods may vary, some general time management principles include:

- Writing down all of the tasks one needs to accomplish. Lisa was first instructed to write down everything she needed or wanted to do, both immediately and in the future.
- Prioritizing tasks. After Lisa had constructed her list, the therapist reviewed each item with her, asking questions such as, "How important is this item to you?" "Does this task need to get done right now, or can it be done later?" The therapist suggested that Lisa was trying to do too many things in a short period of time, and as a result, finished very few tasks. Lisa expressed an aversion to what she called "procrastination;" however, the therapist reframed this by suggesting that putting off or delegating less important tasks was not only acceptable, in some cases it was critical.
- Scheduling. Lisa did not keep a personal calendar; as a result, she often felt confused about what to do next. The therapist instructed her to buy a pocket date book that had room to write tasks for each day, as well as a blank area for each week in which she could write additional tasks she needed to accomplish. The therapist worked with Lisa to create a "to do" list for the week, and then broke these tasks down by day. Lisa was instructed to cross each item off of her list when it was finished. Many of our patients have benefited from purchasing hand-held computers that they can synchronize with their home or work computers.
- Using time efficiently. One of the key sources of Lisa's inefficiency was the fact that she spent time at work talking to friends and family on the telephone. The therapist asked Lisa to monitor how much time she spent in this activity; Lisa was surprised to discover that she spent nearly two hours (one quarter of her work day) making personal telephone calls. The therapist suggested she refrain from using the telephone for reasons other than business while at work, and to call her friends and family from home in the evening. This principle relates to the stimulus control procedures described in Chapter 8.
- Making time for recreation, relaxation, and exercise. Lisa was initially amused by the therapist's suggestion that she actually write a 10-minute break into her work schedule. However, she was willing to do so and found that she felt clearer and more energized afterward. The therapist also instructed her to schedule a daily evening walk around the neighborhood with her children.

CHAPTER 13

CHANGING YOUR THINKING:

Module 3: Cognitive Restructuring

As we have mentioned above and other researchers have stated explicitly, cognitive factors are thought to play at least some role in the conceptualization of TTM, although generally speaking it appears that this role is not a central one (Franklin et al., 2006; Stanley & Cohen, 1999). It may be the case, however, that the heterogeneity of TTM presentation in general obscures the more critical role that cognition plays in TTM for a subset of patients. For example, Christenson et al. (1994) examined different pulling styles in a large clinical sample of adults with TTM and were able to identify a subset of patients whose pulling was more "focused" and associated with affective states such as the desire to achieve "evenness" or to remove certain kinds of hairs deemed unacceptable such as coarse hairs, gray hairs, etc.; recent data from the web-based, large-scale Trichotillomania Impact Study in adults provided additional support for this position that some individuals with TTM pull in order to alleviate anxiety or other negative affective states (Flessner et al., 2006). Thus cognition may play an important predictive role in the pulling behavior for such patients. We have also encountered in our clinical practices some individuals with TTM who clearly identify cognitive precursors to pulling that have to do with patient's expectations about the effects of pulling: "If I pull a few now I'll calm down and then I'll be able to go back into the meeting." From a clinical standpoint, then, it is important to identify these precursors as part of the awareness training process, and it may also be necessary in such cases to provide such patient with cognitive strategies to combat these dysfunctional thoughts. If you encounter such patients in practice, the techniques laid out in this chapter may very well prove helpful in reducing affective distress resulting from such thoughts and thereby weaken urges to pull.

WHAT IS COGNITIVE RESTRUCTURING?

We anticipate that many clinicians who are interested in TTM treatment have already had at least some exposure to cognitive theories of psychopathology, cognitive therapy, and cognitive restructuring, which is a technique that is often used in cognitive therapy. Cognitive therapies now have a long history of use in the field of clinical psychology and psychiatry, with key developers including Aaron T. Beck, Albert Ellis, William Glasser, and others pioneering a new emphasis on the influence that thinking, distorted or inaccurate thinking in particular, has on emotion and on behavior. The basic premise of these approaches is that dysfunctional beliefs underlie strong negative emotions, which in turn lead to maladaptive behavior, which fuels more negative thinking. Take for example a socially anxious person named Joe who attends a party. Joe might be thinking on the drive over to the party that "Nobody is going to like me" or that "Everyone will find me boring," and these thoughts lead to increased heart rate, sweating, intrusive images of strangers at the party walking away in mid-sentence or doing other such unhelpful things when encountering Joe. The effect of this thinking and these now intense emotions on Joe's behavior might translate behaviorally to driving back home (active avoidance) or entering the house where the party is being held and sitting in a relatively isolated corner (passive avoidance) or, when forced to interact, engaging in other subtle avoidance behaviors such as averting eye contact or providing monosyllabic or other very short answers to questions posed by others to Joe. The likely response to these behaviors is disinterest on the part of the other person or people in the interaction, who might soon be looking for a way to back out of the interaction to find a more active conversational partner. Joe of course receives confirmation of his initial thoughts from these responses, which confirms his beliefs about himself and sets up subsequent difficulties for him at the next social gathering.

Cognitive theories places a central role on the dysfunctional beliefs thought to underlie Joe's thoughts about himself and about people's responses to him, and thus identifying these beliefs is critical to helping Joe modify them, which again according to cognitive theories of psychopathology is necessary for reducing negative emotions and maladaptive behaviors. Thus, cognitive therapists rely on techniques that are designed to first help the patient recognize what they were thinking in problematic situations. Thought records are used in most cognitive therapies to facilitate this process, and although they may differ across types of cognitive therapies (e.g., Rational Emotive Therapy vs. Cognitive Therapy in the Beck school) their purpose is to help the patient begin to challenge the thoughts to see if they hold up to logical scrutiny. Various techniques are used to implement this second step, such as Socratic questioning, the "downward arrow" technique, etc., but their purpose is to help the patient logically evaluate whether the irrational thoughts and their underlying core beliefs can stand a strong empirical test. In our work we have tended to use a "cross-examination" metaphor for our adult patients as a means to help the patient understand that the goal is to poke holes in the logic of these thoughts and beliefs, regardless of whether they felt plausible or realistic at the time. When the logic has been challenged sufficiently, cognitive therapists will often encourage patients to generate a rational response to the initial thought or belief, as a means of teaching the person that just because you think something doesn't necessarily mean it's accurate; this part of the therapy is often referred to as cognitive restructuring. All of these cognitive techniques are taught at first based on situations that have already occurred, but clearly the goal is that the patient becomes more and more efficient with them, such that they can recognize, challenge, and replace such dysfunctional thoughts in real time.

We do not anticipate that a single chapter on cognitive restructuring techniques will create expert cognitive therapists – experience and training will serve that goal. Nevertheless, we wish to include this section on cognitive restructuring because many therapists are already familiar with the methods and use them routinely in their clinical practices with other patients. What we wish to do here is to explicate how such techniques might be used in the context of treating TTM, especially when the functional analysis or ongoing treatment has highlighted the central role that maladaptive thinking is playing in the TTM cycle or in the patient's emotional life more generally speaking, which of course could increase stress and feed back to pulling urges and behavior indirectly.

COGNITION AND TTM

TTM may also be associated with specific irrational beliefs about the pulling itself and its likely effects on other people in the environment, and here again cognitive restructuring techniques may prove useful in reducing affect associated with these cognitions and hence indirectly influence pulling behavior. For example, if a patient has concluded in advance that other people will deem him/her socially unacceptable because of the pulling behavior, he/she would be unlikely to test this hypothesis and hence increase the sense of isolation, suffering, and unfairness of it all, which is unpleasant in and of itself but also may lead back indirectly to increased pulling behavior. Thus, cognitive restructuring techniques may prove useful in encouraging patients to refrain from drawing such negative conclusions in the absence of compelling data from the environment (e.g., public stoning, direct statements about the patient's unacceptability).

Even if cognitive factors in and of themselves are generally thought to be unlikely to lead directly to pulling (Christenson & Mansueto, 1999), there is an extensive literature available on the role that cognition plays in the development and maintenance of affective and other emotional disorders (see Reineke et al., 2003). Moreover, the presence of intense and unremitting negative affect may *indirectly* lead to increased urges to pull, even if there is not a direct pathway from cognition to pulling evident in most TTM patients. Thus, if self-monitoring data suggests that depression, anxiety, and anger typically precedes pulling in a given patient, then cognitive techniques may prove to be useful adjuncts in "shutting off one of the valves" that fuels pulling. Cognitive techniques devoted to identifying, critically evaluating, and correcting mistaken beliefs represent the core interventions for most of the empirically supported protocols, and their specific application to TTM is demonstrated below; cognitive restructuring sheets are also provided in the Appendix.

It is our position that cognitive restructuring may therefore play a potentially important role in the treatment of at least some patients with TTM. We advocate integrating CR techniques into a protocol that still includes emphasis on the core elements described in Section 2 of the book. Clinical judgment needs to be used to determine whether the cognitive techniques being incorporated are useful in this adjunctive role, and if not the decision might be made to switch more formally to a cognitive approach. Here this would result in skating on the thinner end of the empirical pond, since as yet there have been no controlled studies of cognitive restructuring alone in the treatment of TTM. This caveat notwithstanding, clinicians should exercise judgment as to best reduce the effects of the identified negative cognitions on the clinical management of TTM. If it is clear that a secondary comorbid diagnosis has developed or has become more prominent in treatment, the reader is referred to the chapter on the clinical management of comorbidity.

It is evident from a developmental perspective that thinking in adults is not the same as thinking in teenagers and in young children, and this reality needs to be taken into consideration if a clinician has identified with a younger patient the presence of negative, persistent, and affectively intense cognitions, whether they impact on TTM directly or not. This may be especially true for teenagers with TTM, given that so much emphasis is placed in adolescent culture on acceptance and fitting in with an identified peer group, a task that is at the very least complicated by the presence of a disorder in which the effects are often evident to others. Here again, cognitive restructuring techniques might prove useful, although it is imperative to tailor their use to the cognitive abilities and developmental stage of the patient. Very young children may not be developmentally ready to introspect and pay careful attention to what is happening cognitively, and thus generally speaking the younger the child, the more adaptation will be needed to make these techniques applicable. We provide several clinical examples of such adaptations in this chapter, but the interested reader who wishes to know more about the developmental literature on this topic and on the sorts of adaptations likely to be helpful for children and adolescents is referred to Kendall's (2006) text on CBT procedures for children and adolescents, particularly to the opening chapter by Kendall (2006) and a chapter on treating adolescents specifically by Holmbeck et al. (2006).

Below, we provide examples of the use of cognitively-based treatment techniques for TTM. Such discussions can be facilitated by encouraging patients to track their negative thinking on sheets like those included in the Appendix, but often in clinical circumstances the opportunity to help a patient identify, evaluate, and modify dysfunctional thinking that is contributing directly or indirectly to TTM can occur in the context of discussions of other topics and techniques, and hence might arise "on the fly." It may be that when conversations in sessions are leading routinely to discussion of irrational beliefs that directly or indirectly influence pulling, the therapist might consider using the CR module and being more formal in incorporating these techniques into the treatment. Below we have provided clinical examples of using CR techniques with a patient whose pulling is directly influenced by cognition. Moreover, because there are important developmental differences between adults and youth with respect to use of cognitive techniques, we have also included an example of CR with a child as well, with firm grounding in a collaborative problem-solving approach.

COGNITIVE RESTRUCTURING WITH AN ADULT: TTM-RELATED COGNITIONS

T: So I see that you've got your Thought Records with you – how were they to use?

P: It was hard to remember to do it at first, but I think I learned something from them anyway.

T: What did you learn?

P: Well like we were saying last week it seems like the way I am thinking about the pulling is not always so helpful, and might be leading me to pull more.

T: Can you give me some examples from your sheet this week?

P: Yeah, from an episode I tracked the other night I learned that the things I was telling myself before I pulled probably led me to get started sooner, and then my thinking right after that same episode probably led me to feel really badly and keep pulling for longer.

T: That sounds really useful – can you first walk me through the thoughts you were having before that pulling episode started? Where were you?

P: I was home alone after work, sitting in the living room with the TV on.

T: What did you notice in your thinking?

P: *I was focusing on the events of the day, how stressed I was feeling, and then I remember thinking, "I had a really tough day – I deserve to pull at least some."*

T: *From what you've told me that's not the way it usually works for you – what you've typically described is zoning out in front of the TV after work and then noticing you've been pulling.*

P: *That's true, but this time it was really clear that I was giving myself permission to pull because the day had been so crappy.*

T: *And there was also something else in there, wasn't there?*

P: *You mean the "at least some" part?*

T: *Right – like you're telling yourself it's OK to pull at least some when you've had a tough day, but that once you cross over past "at least some" then it becomes bad again.*

P: *Right.*

T: *I wonder whether you have a really clear definition in your head of what "some" means?*

P: *(Pauses) Well, in this case I defined "some" as being slightly less than what I actually pulled.*

T: *Meaning that you exceeded the amount you deserved to pull?*

P: *Right.*

T: *Do you know if this is how it usually works for you when you tell yourself that you're allowed to pull some?*

P: *Now that you mention it, I think I usually wind up concluding that I pulled more than some.*

T: *Regardless of the actual number or amount of time?*

P: *Yeah, usually.*

T: *And when this happens – when you violate the rule you set for yourself – what does that lead to?*

P: *In this case it led to pretty intense sadness and lots of negative thinking that I wrote down on the sheet.*

T: *And did you notice any effects on pulling when all that came up?*

P: *Sure – more pulling, and for lots longer than usual during that time period after work.*

T: *So the initial thinking about how you deserved to pull because of the day you'd had led you to try to handle the stress with pulling, but then once you violated the rule about pulling "more than some", whatever that means, it led to a spiral of negative affect, more dysfunctional thinking, and more pulling?*

P: *Right.*

T: So with that in mind, how might you respond the next time you have that thought about deserving to pull at least some?

P: Well I have to see that for what it is, which is a strategy for handling stress that leads to more stress, and I have to tell myself that I don't deserve to suffer like that.

T: Nice. Is that what you wrote in the Rational Response column of your sheet?

P: Something like that, although not quite so clearly – it helps me still to discuss it in here.

T: Sure – you're only now getting used to paying attention to your dysfunctional thinking and in talking back to it, so it won't seem so natural just yet. If you keep at this though it will become more reflexive and you'll be able to do it successfully in real time, which means you'll be less likely to let the negative thinking get away from you and then wind up paying for it later.

P: That sounds good – it does seem a little weird still now.

T: It will get easier to do, though, trust me. Now let's look at the cognitions that followed the violation of the "at least some" rule. What did you write down on your sheet?

P: Well I noticed that once I decided that I'd pulled more than I should have, I started really berating myself.

T: The specifics are probably important – what did you say?

P: (Hesitates) I told myself that I was a bad person, weak, and that I should be able to handle stress like regular people instead of resorting to pulling.

T: Pretty heavy stuff. What was its effect on your mood?

P: (Chuckles) It wasn't very good, I'll tell you that!

T: And yet it stays in your lexicon, probably because you're just not used to noticing it and talking back to it.

P: Right – I've paid a lot more attention to my thinking in the last several weeks, and I can see that the negative litany of recrimination and blame isn't making my job easier.

T: Like a big sack of rocks, really. So you were telling yourself that you were a bad person because you violated the rule, weak, and that you should be able to handle work stress differently.

P: Right.

T: When I see "shoulds" in people's automatic thoughts I usually start looking for the usual affective result of that kind of thinking, which is guilt. Did you notice that you were feeling guilty about having pulled then?

P: Very guilty.

T: *And what did you come up with for a rational response for that stuff, to take the edge off and minimize the effect of this kind of thinking on your feelings about yourself and about your fight against TTM?*

P: *Well I wrote that I have an illness, and that having an illness doesn't make me a bad person.*

T: *And what was the effect of working that out?*

P: *I felt much better about it then – it's like I'm cutting myself some slack, getting away from just yelling at myself, and getting towards doing something more constructive instead of just feeling bad about myself.*

T: *Sounds pretty productive. Did that translate into action in any way?*

P: *Well the next day after yet another crappy day at work I decided that I should go get dinner out instead of going straight home and sitting in the same place feeling the same way that I did the night before.*

T: *Terrific – so the cognitive restructuring stuff helped you to implement stimulus control more effectively.*

P: *I guess it did – I can't say that I thought of it quite so formally, but I figured that it just made more sense to go be somewhere that I wouldn't be quite so vulnerable.*

T: *Good thinking. Did you go alone or did you go with a coworker?*

P: *Actually I went with a co-worker, and I even asked her if she wanted to go out – not my usual thing.*

T: *Someone you know pretty well?*

P: *(Smiles) Nope, not even – just somebody who's new to our office and to the city; she seems nice and she's kinda quiet like me so I thought it wouldn't be too intimidating.*

T: *Great – and it went OK?*

P: *Yeah, really well – she's not used to the toxic environment in our place and so I think she found it helpful to talk to someone about it who's been there for a while – I gave her the scoop, and we are going to see a movie at some point soon.*

T: *Terrific – I know that this was a goal of yours down the road, too.*

P: *Maybe not so far down the road, and obviously a better way to handle stress than sitting at home alone.*

T: *It sounds like you found the CR stuff helpful – you should probably continue to monitor your thinking since I'm sure there are many more rocks to look under for evidence that you're not being very kind to yourself, and the effect of that seems to be more negative emotion, isolating yourself, and probably more pulling.*

P: *I think you're right about that.*

COGNITIVE RESTRUCTURING/PROBLEM SOLVING WITH A CHILD

T: So as I go over your monitoring stuff here it seems like there was a pretty big spike in pulling late Saturday afternoon. You were at home?

P: Yeah, I went straight to my room after the first day of softball practice and just started pulling.

T: It sounds like you knew you were pulling that time.

P: Oh, yeah, I knew – I was really upset, and just trying to calm myself down before I had to come back down for dinner and the company we were having.

T: Do you remember why you were that upset?

P: Yeah, it was because I was assigned to a new team this year without my best friend, which was bad enough, but I found out on the first day that the kids on the new team were really, really mean.

T: So you expected you'd be with your friend again?

P: My mom requested that, and they just didn't do it – they're so stupid!

T: Did you know that before Saturday?

P: Yeah, and they said they couldn't do anything about – I found out last week.

T: That sounds pretty tough – you were expecting to play together again and figured that would make it more fun. Now tell me about the new kids – your age?

P: Mostly, but some of them are older – they moved me up but didn't move my friend up, so she's playing with kids our age or younger.

T: Is that part of why it was hard?

P: Maybe.

T: Older girls – do you expect them to be less friendly?

P: Not always, but these ones were awful – they just looked at me like I was some kind of freak!

T: Was this when people were being introduced to each other?

P: No, before then – I got there early and went to the field where we were supposed to go, and some of them were already there. I just hate them, and I don't want to play this year!

T: Sounds like it wasn't any fun at all, huh? Did you like it last year?

P: I did, especially at the end of the season.

T: How come at the end?

P: Well I was new to this league last year, and I hardly knew anybody.

T: I thought you said your best friend was on the team.

P: She was, but I didn't know her until the season got started.

T: *You met her at softball?*

P: *Yeah, she doesn't go to my school – she goes to Catholic school.*

T: *But you got to know her pretty well I see.*

P: *Yeah, we went to the pool last summer almost every day together, did sleep-overs, that kind of stuff. She's nice, and she's into a lot of stuff that I'm into.*

T: *Like?*

P: *Softball, other sports, horses, and this show called Saddle Club – most kids don't know it, but we're really into it, so we play it a lot together.*

T: *That sounds like a lot of fun – you'll still get to do that anyway, right?*

P: *Sure – softball's only one practice a week and one game every weekend, and they're all at the same field.*

T: *So you'll probably be able to go there together still, just wind up at different diamonds?*

P: *Right – our Moms are friends now too, so they'll probably switch with the driving.*

T: *That would be nice – a friendly face to see before and after you go.*

P: *I just wish we could play together again, though.*

T: *Sure – makes sense. Now let's go back to the new kids – do you know any of them?*

P: *No – only to see them around. They're not from my school either.*

T: *So bring me back to the field on Saturday so I can understand this better – you walked up to a group of them, but I don't remember if you told me how many.*

P: *There were four of them.*

T: *Did they know each other?*

P: *They seemed to – they were paired off and playing catch.*

T: *You mean when you walked up to them?*

P: *Right.*

T: *So they were already doing something.*

P: *Yeah.*

T: *When you saw that what did you do?*

P: *I just stood there and waited for somebody to invite me to play catch.*

T: *Did you say anything?*

P: *No, I just looked at them for a while and then I started putting on my cleats – I was already mad about not playing with my friend, and when they didn't invite me to catch I got even madder.*

T: *What did they do?*

P: Nothing – they just played catch.

T: And what were you doing?

P: I was fixing my laces and looking down at the ground.

T: For how long?

P: Not too long – the coach came and called us into the dugout.

T: Did you go?

P: I did, after a minute or so.

T: Still pretty mad at that point?

P: Yeah, I kept thinking about how much fun last year's team was and how much this year's team was going to stink.

T: You mean because you didn't know anybody and they didn't say anything to you?

P: Right, but last year's team we laughed and joked around all the time.

T: I have an idea – do you want to play a little game right here and now?

P: What kind of game?

T: It's like a detective game – let's pretend that a new law has just been passed and you and I are given the responsibility to enforce it. The new law is that you're not allowed to be mean to people, and if you are mean you can be arrested. Why don't you and I see if we can get enough evidence together to see if these kids from softball could be arrested for breaking that new law.

P: That sounds good – should be easy!

T: Maybe so, but remember, we need enough evidence for the judge to convict them, so we're going to have to gather a lot of information before we go arresting anybody.

P: OK.

T: Let's start with the obvious stuff first – you can arrest somebody for being super mean if they hit somebody on purpose for no reason – that seems like it would be part of the law, right?

P: Right.

T: So let's see: did any of these four kids hit you, or anybody else, on purpose for no reason?

P: No.

T: You sure, detective? We don't want to miss any really big pieces of evidence.

P: Nope, I'm sure.

T: What about hitting somebody by accident? Did they do any of that?

P: No.

T: Spitting on them?

P: No.

T: Setting fire to their softball gloves?

P: (Chuckles) No – I would have remembered that.

T: OK, so no hitting on purpose, no hitting by accident, no spitting, and no fires, right?

P: Right.

T: OK then, so let's look at some other things that they might have done or said that would violate the new law and let us arrest them once and for all.

P: They didn't say anything to me the whole time I was there before the coach came.

T: Well that rules out that they said something super-mean, but maybe we're onto something else then. Did they say anything super-mean?

P: No, they didn't say anything.

T: OK then, let's look at what they didn't do.

P: They didn't say hello.

T: Even after you spoke up and said hello to them?

P: Well, no, I didn't do that.

T: So you didn't say hello and they didn't say hello, do I have it right?

P: Right.

T: And what were they doing when you got there?

P: Playing catch.

T: So they weren't just looking right at you when you came up.

P: (Hesitates) No, they were watching the ball. They all throw kind of hard, too, so they had to watch the ball.

T: And after a few minutes you looked down and put on your cleats, right? What were they doing at that time?

P: Still playing catch.

T: Did other kids come up during that time too?

P: Yeah, a few.

T: And what did the Gang of Four do when these kids came up?

P: Nothing, I think – they just kept on throwing.

T: What did those other kids do then?

P: Some went down where the coach was, a few sat near me and put on their cleats, too.

T: *So these kids didn't treat you any differently than the other kids?*

P: *No, I guess not.*

T: *And how long were you there?*

P: *Not too long.*

T: *You said the coach came out and called you all in?*

P: *Right.*

T: *Did they go?*

P: *Right away.*

T: *How about you?*

P: *I waited for a minute.*

T: *And when did you get up and go towards the dugout?*

P: *After one of the players came back a bit and told me that the lady with the batbag was our coach.*

T: *Was it one of the Gang of Four, or was it a different player?*

P: *No, it was one of the four.*

T: *Did she say it in a supermean way, so we could arrest her for that?*

P: *No, she said it regular.*

T: *Like she wanted you to know something important?*

P: *Yeah, so I wouldn't just keep sitting there.*

T: *Did she wait for you to get up or did she just turn around and run away from you?*

P: *No she waited, and when I reached her she ran in with me.*

T: *Trip you with a bat?*

P: *(Laughs) No, she didn't do anything bad.*

T: *So Detective, it sounds like we're going to have to let her go, huh?*

P: *I guess we do – she wasn't super mean, and maybe she was even a little bit friendly. I still don't know why they didn't say hello.*

T: *Let's go back and look at that again – maybe there's some evidence we can gather about that. You said that you didn't know any of them, and they didn't know you, right?*

P: *Right.*

T: *So they couldn't use your name and say hi because they didn't know your name.*

P: *Yeah.*

T: *And they were in the middle of a game of catch?*

P: *Two games of catch – two balls, two girls each one.*

T: *So there was a lot to keep an eye on.*

P: *Yeah, but I think they saw me.*

T: *Did you say anything to them?*

P: *No, I just sat there.*

T: *So you didn't say anything to them, and they didn't say anything to you.*

P: *Right.*

T: *Do we have good evidence to convict them yet?*

P: *No, not really.*

T: *You asked a good question earlier that we should think about now. Are there any other explanations for why they didn't say hi besides that they're all super mean?*

P: *Well, they were playing catch already, and I didn't say anything to them – I just felt awkward.*

T: *Is it possible that they weren't sure how to handle it either?*

P: *I guess, but they were talking to each other.*

T: *But you said you found out that they all knew each other from last year's team, right? Could that be why it was easier for them to talk to each other but not to you?*

P: *Probably.*

T: *If you were there with three of your teammates from last year and a new girl came up like you did, would you find it easier to talk to your friends or to the new kid?*

P: *My friends.*

T: *I wonder if that might have been what happened here?*

P: *Maybe, they did say bye when we all left at the end of practice.*

T: *So it's possible that the hard part at the beginning had more to do with not knowing each other yet, rather than with them being super mean?*

P: *Yeah, I see that now.*

T: *Good – it will be important to check that out this week. How could you do that?*

P: *I could say hi to them at the beginning and see what happens.*

T: *Do you remember the start of last year's season? You mentioned how great it was at the end, but do you remember if it started out great?*

P: *Actually, I remember that it was a little weird at first, too.*

T: *But it got easier as you got to know each other, right?*

P: *Right.*

T: Is it possible that this could be true of this year, too?

P: Maybe, but I still wish my best friend was on my team again.

T: Yeah, that's unfortunate, but maybe you could make some friends here too, and then they could meet your best friend since you're all interested in softball. Who knows, maybe somebody on your team is into Saddle Club too.

P: You think?

T: Maybe. How would you find out?

P: I could ask.

T: You could also ask about horses, since people who are into horses might like Saddle Club.

P: Yeah, and then I could tell them about it and we could expand our fan club!

T: Good thinking – you think you can try this again this week trying to keep that Detective idea in mind – make sure you have good evidence before you come to any conclusions?

P: Yeah, I think it would help.

T: And if softball wasn't so upsetting this week, maybe Saturday won't be such a tough day for pulling.

P: I sure hope so.

CHAPTER 14

WHEN OTHER PROBLEMS ARE ALSO PRESENT:

Module 4: Clinical Management of Comorbid Problems

MANAGEMENT OF PSYCHIATRIC COMORBIDITY: A CHALLENGE TO CLINICIANS

As we described earlier in the book, TTM in adults is associated with significant psychiatric comorbidity in adults (e.g., Christenson et al., 1991a), to the point where it appears that Axis I and/or Axis II comorbidity is likely to be the rule rather than the exception. The data that have been gathered thus far in youth seeking clinical services suggest that, although comorbidity does appear to be less common in youth than in adults, it is not at all unusual for TTM to co-occur with other psychiatric problems (e.g., Tolin et al., 2006). Thus, clinicians who treat TTM and related disorders must assess and manage comorbidity, regardless of whether their practices are focused on adults or children and adolescents.

As we see it, one of the core challenges facing clinicians is whether and how best to manage psychiatric comorbidity in the context of providing treatment for a specific disorder such as TTM. There are several potentially reasonable options to consider in the face of comorbidity, each of which will be considered below: 1) continue to focus on TTM symptoms regardless of the presence of symptoms of other disorders; 2) attempt to incorporate some clinical procedures and session time to manage the symptoms of the co-occurring disorder but continue to keep the focus on TTM; 3) shift the focus of treatment to the management of the comorbid problem(s); and 4) refer for specialty services to handle the comorbid symptoms, and suspend TTM treatment until those symptoms are under better control. Clearly none of these options is going to fit every case, and the expertise of the clinician will dictate in part whether the latter two options are even viable. Below we discuss each of these in turn, and provide suggestions as to how one might arrive at a decision as to which option is the best fit for specific clinical circumstances.

OPTION 1: CONTINUE TO FOCUS ON TTM

When a patient enters treatment for TTM, a functional analysis of the pattern of pulling for that specific individual might be one place where evidence of the potential effects of comorbid conditions will be uncovered. For example, detailed questioning about situations that typically result in pulling might reveal that social anxiety plays a regular and significant role in the development and intensity of urges to pull, such that these symptoms are actually a regular precipitant of pulling. Presumably the patient in this case has identified TTM as a target of treatment, or such a functional analysis would not have commenced. In light of information about this patient's pulling and social anxiety, the clinician must discuss the observation with the patient and consider whether a continued focus on TTM would be best, or whether a shift to working on social anxiety disorder symptoms would be better. Patient preference is thus a good place to start in considering whether the continued focus on TTM is the most appropriate action to take; the link to motivation here is clear, and patient motivation to reduce pulling is a critical component of any successful treatment approach to TTM. If the patient sees another agenda that is more important to address, the success of a focus on TTM will necessarily be limited.

Patient preference notwithstanding, the intensity and functional impairment associated with both disorders is also important to consider: using our example of comorbid social phobia symptoms above, if that patient reports that TTM is the problem that is causing the most distress, then the clinician might be best off continuing the focus there and use the presence of difficult social situations and the associated anxiety symptoms as "early warning signs" for the implementation of TTM treatment procedures, such as making sure that "fiddle toy baskets" are ready and fully stocked in the weeks prior to attending a major social function that is likely to temporarily increase anxiety and urges to pull. We encourage clinicians to at least consider a continued focus on TTM primarily when the TTM-related impairment is high and the comorbid symptoms are not extremely severe or causing a great deal of separate functional impairment. Moreover, if there is a strong functional link between TTM and the secondary problem, moving off TTM and towards the other problem(s) might result in a lost opportunity to get two birds with one stone. In the case example raised above, if anxiety in social situations is exacerbated by fears that the patient will be "found out" as being a hairpuller, then teaching the patient how to successfully manage and then reduce pulling behavior and urges to pull will likely have a positive effect on social anxiety as well.

Option 2: Attempt to Focus Some Treatment Time on Comorbidity but with the Intention of Moving Back to TTM.

Our second option involves a temporary shift of focus away from TTM and towards the comorbid problem(s), but with an explicit intention to return the focus of treatment as soon as this is feasible clinically. This sort of approach has been implemented in the context of an ongoing multi-site clinical trial in pediatric OCD on which one of us (MEF) serves as a site Principal Investigator. The procedure used in that study is known as Adjunctive Services and Attrition Prevention, or ASAP. ASAP procedures have been employed in multiple pediatric treatment outcome studies (e.g., Pediatric OCD Treatment Study, 2004; Treatment of Adolescent Depression Study Team, 2005). Among its primary purposes is the goal of providing clinicians with a way to manage emergent clinical problems that extend beyond those associated with the primary disorder, but without substantially violating the treatment protocol. For example, during treatment for a primary clinical condition, symptoms associated with a secondary disorder occasionally become more prominent during the acute treatment phase, necessitating clinical decisions about whether it is in the patient's best interest to continue with treatment for the primary identified condition, and, if so, how best to handle these new symptoms. The ASAP procedure allows for up to two additional sessions during the standard treatment protocol to provide the clinician the opportunity to stem the tide; if these sessions are judged to be inadequate on clinical grounds (e.g., development of a serious major depressive episode), then the study team would recommend that the standard treatment protocol be replaced with open treatment that will allow for even greater attention to the more prominent features of the emergent symptoms (for a detailed review of an ASAP protocol see Franklin, Foa, & March, 2003).

Underlying the rationale for inclusion of ASAP procedures are two fundamental clinical judgments. The first of these is the belief that it is imperative to try to maintain focus on the primary disorder when feasible and when in the patient's best interest. The risk of not doing so is to dissipate efforts and allow treatment to devolve into a "crisis du jour" mode, which necessarily waters down the delivery of the intended protocol for the primary problem. The second of these judgments is that although it is important to at least attempt to maintain focus on the primary disorder, it is also imperative to be sufficiently flexible in the presence of emergent symptoms and problems.

To demonstrate this approach using a specific case example, consider the presence of comorbid depressive symptoms that may warrant a brief intervention with the intention of returning the focus of treatment back to TTM. As discussed previously, depression and anxiety problems are both quite common in individuals with TTM, and may have some shared and some unique pathways by which they influence pulling. Depression is often exacerbated by stress, and hence any predictably stressful situations (e.g., work deadlines, finals week, relationship difficulties) should be viewed as times when these pre-existing internalizing symptoms might be on the rise and thus likely to result in increased urges to pull. Thus, we often ask our patients in the last part of our sessions whether they have anything important or stressful coming up that might influence the urges in the coming week; with patients who have identified comorbid symptoms such as depression, this inquiry also includes attention to the ways that the known stressor might affect depression. From there, it is important to discuss with the patient whether he/she has already identified strategies that are effective in reducing the comorbid depressive symptoms or, alternatively, noticed responses to feeling depressed that tend to exacerbate mood problems. One such example is from an adult patient who noticed that when she becomes depressed she tends to isolate herself from friends and family, which in turn results in worsening symptoms of both depression and TTM. With this patient it was important to identify this pattern and plan in advance to circumvent the problem using behavioral activation strategies such as scheduling pleasurable activities with friends and family regardless of motivation level. The increased activity level during a time when depressive symptoms were increasing served to prevent an exacerbation of depression, but it also had an indirect effect on TTM in that the patient reported that time alone when feeling depressed was a risk factor for increased urges and for cognitions such as "Why bother resisting – it won't matter anyway," which of course tended to be associated with decreased use of monitoring, stimulus control and competing response strategies. Implementation of this additional strategy may take only one or two devoted sessions and regular follow-up on the efficacy of these interventions, but the goal would be to add such strategies to the patient's repertoire and then return the focus to teaching and implementing TTM-specific strategies.

Anxiety symptoms also play a key role in the psychopathology of many patients with TTM, and therefore need to be taken into account in the development of a treatment plan. Data from our study with youth suggested that GAD was the most common comorbid diagnosis. GAD is characterized by uncontrollable and frequent worries, often in relation to a wide variety of topics, and typically includes associated physical symptoms such as muscle tension, GI symptoms, sleep disturbance, and fatigue. Because these latter symptoms may trigger urges to pull, it is important to query patients who have this comorbidity about whether they have identified ways to manage their worries successfully. In some cases, it might be useful to spend a session or two presenting a conceptualization of GAD and worry to the patient, and including some formal cognitive techniques and instruction in recognizing worries for what they are and allowing them to come and go without getting actively engaged with them (i.e., cultivating detached observation of worry content) in order to help the patient gain some increased mastery over worry and, by extension, over the effects of worry on urges to pull. Occasionally patients with comorbid GAD worry in an uncontrolled manner about the implementation of TTM treatment procedures (e.g., "what if I'm not doing the competing response training the right way?"), a tendency which requires discussion up front about the inherent flexibility of the program and the "trial and error" approach we wish to encourage as patients figure out with the help of the therapist what techniques and strategies will work best for them in reducing pulling. If this attempt to circumvent worry does not prove helpful, again it may be time to devote a session or two to helping the patient identify such worries, generate specific rational responses to them, and/or to implementing distancing techniques (e.g., imagine your worries as words melting over a hot fire) designed to improve perceived control over worry.

Another common comorbidity that can complicate treatment for TTM or related problems is alcohol or other substance abuse. Christenson and colleagues, as well as other investigators, have found that individuals with TTM are at increased risk for these kinds of comorbid problems, and there is evidence that a subset of individuals with TTM specifically use alcohol or other drugs to reduce urges to pull (Woods et al., 2006). One of us (MEF) once treated a college student with TTM who tended to have a significant increase in pulling behavior on Friday, Saturday, and Sunday mornings relative to the rest of her week. Early monitoring of academic stress and demands did not reveal any discernable pattern or reliable predictors, but an offhand comment made by the patient about upcoming weekend party plans clued therapist and patient alike into the possibility that hangovers following episodes of binge drinking were actually predicting these regular increases in pulling urges. An experiment was planned in which the patient would use common controlled drinking strategies (e.g., alternating between alcoholic drinks and 24 oz. glasses of water) to determine whether this suspected relationship was indeed explaining the morning pulling. It turned out that this was indeed the case, and the treatment focus expanded temporarily to include strategies designed to reduce binge drinking as a means to reduce the after-effects on pulling urges and resistance to such urges, but also as an important goal in and of itself. The fine-tuning of the controlled drinking strategies in this case took only about two more focused sessions, and the patient's relatively benign drinking history and ability to successfully implement these strategies without any withdrawal symptoms suggested that the treatment could then be refocused on TTM, albeit with new information about the role that alcohol abuse played for this patient in urges to pull. In circumstances such as this, the success of the chosen clinical strategies for reducing drinking allowed the treatment to remain focused primarily on TTM; if an intervention of this sort proves unsuccessful, then the treatment plan itself may need to be revisited and the treatment refocused on alcohol abuse. In the case discussed above the outcome was not clear until the experiment was attempted; clearly, though, if the alcohol abuse was more pronounced and associated with greater impairment than the TTM, then the focus on TTM would need to be reconsidered. We discuss this important point in greater detail below.

OPTION 3: SHIFT THE FOCUS OF TREATMENT TO THE COMORBID PROBLEM.

The first two of our four suggestions about clinical management of comorbidity involved making concerted efforts to maintain the focus of treatment on TTM. We recognize, however, that this approach is not always preferable. The severity of the comorbid symptoms, associated functional impairment, the patient's history, presence of suicidality or homicidality, emergence or re-emergence of symptoms of thought disorder or mania, and other such considerations would necessitate use of an alternative strategy of shifting the treatment to the comorbid problems. Let us return again to an example of comorbid depression, but in a case in which the symptoms of depression are considerably more serious and the patient's history of major depressive episodes more clear. In our work we have occasionally encountered patients with such histories who believe at the beginning of treatment that the depression is under sufficient control that a focus on TTM is warranted; sometimes, however, the depressive symptoms worsen over the course of time, and get to the point where they become the primary problem. Patients who are ordinarily compliant with self-monitoring and implementing stimulus control and competing response strategies who begin to demonstrate consistent problems doing what they have already learned how to do might be suffering from a relapse of MDD; this is another reason why we routinely administer depression monitoring scales on a weekly basis in treatment (e.g., DASS-21, Beck Depression Inventory) and encourage therapists to do the same, especially with patients with such histories. Examination of these scales and frank discussion with the patient about their meaning, clinical interview of the patient about current depressive symptoms, consideration of the patient's explanations for why compliance for TTM procedures has decreased (e.g., "Because none of this matters any more – I'm only going to be unhappy anyway") are all useful data to help answer the question of whether it would be in the patient's best interests to shift the focus of treatment to the increasing depressive symptoms. In this case therapists will have to use their best judgment as to whether they are qualified to administer effective treatment for the comorbid depression and, if so, a new treatment plan should be discussed and agreed to with the patient.

Substance abuse is another common problem that can take the focus of treatment away from TTM for more than a brief period of time. If we consider the case example above of the college student whose binge drinking episodes often resulted in hangovers and the hangovers predicted increased difficulty with TTM, the therapist should take care to conduct a careful assessment of current alcohol use, history of use and abuse, prior inpatient or outpatient detoxification, family history of alcoholism, and other factors to determine whether a temporary shift will be sufficient. In the case above this proved to be the case; however, we have both encountered situations in our clinical practices where the substance abuse/dependence is too pronounced or the attempts to reduce drinking too ineffective to be able to turn attention back to the TTM. We have encountered cases clinically in which cocaine use has exacerbated TTM, and when monitoring sheets have been modified to examine the cocaine use specifically it has become evident within a short period of time that the cocaine use has been both heavy and daily. Accordingly, the recommendation in such situations would be to turn the clinical attention to reducing cocaine use, leaving the TTM treatment aside until the cocaine problem had been reduced and sobriety maintained for at least several months. Again, whether this treatment can be spearheaded by the treating clinician depends in large part on their expertise and the severity and impairment of the substance abuse problem.

We have also encountered situations in which trauma history and associated PTSD symptoms have compromised acute TTM treatment, and thus merited clinical attention instead. For example, we have each treated patients whose pulling appears to be much more prominent when at home alone at night; this is not unusual in TTM in general, but investigation of what the patient makes of this increase is important. In one such case, the patient described these times of the day as "scary," both because of the fear of break-ins, but also because she was less occupied with her work at that time and thus more vulnerable to intrusive recollections of her sexual abuse experiences. The patient had revealed the trauma history up front but did not meet criteria for PTSD at the time of intake; rather, the process of monitoring her thinking and trying to become more aware of the situations and thoughts that triggered pulling had drawn her attention to this pattern, and a recent stranger rape in her neighborhood and the associated news coverage had exacerbated symptoms of hyperarousal and avoidance, which are hallmarks of PTSD. In this case the patient and therapist agreed to focus on the PTSD instead, and a course of Prolonged Exposure was recommended. The therapist in this case referred to a female colleague because the patient had reported a preference for treatment by a woman for the sexual abuse symptoms; the expertise of the therapist and the preference of the patient may dictate shifting the therapy but not the therapist in other cases.

OPTION 4: REFER FOR SPECIALTY SERVICES

When a shift of clinical attention from TTM to the comorbid problem is deemed appropriate clinically, the therapist must consider whether to keep the case or to refer for other help. A number of factors go into making this decision, including therapist training and experience, the context in which the therapist works (e.g., general outpatient setting vs. impulse control specialty clinic), the extent of work conducted thus far by the therapist and patient together, patient preferences, and the ability of the therapist to provide sufficient clinical care, coverage, and follow-up for the comorbid problem. Clinically we have each had cases in which we have referred out for these other services and other cases in which we have treated "in house;" no discernable pattern has emerged to inform us as to which of these strategies has proven more efficacious for the comorbid problem, although the eventual return to TTM treatment has certainly been higher in the latter case. In the absence of compelling data to inform us either way then about which course is likely best, we encourage clinicians to use their judgment about what to do when the comorbidity proves more than what can be handled while still maintaining a focus on TTM.

CLINICAL CASE EXAMPLE

Below we discuss a case in which the clinician and the therapist ultimately decided to shift attention from TTM to the comorbid condition in midstream rather than to try to stay in the TTM protocol per se. We use the case vignette to provide a more specific example of how to query patients about their comorbid symptoms, and how to arrive at a judgment about the best course of action.

T: So how was the week?

P: Pretty tough, actually, pretty tough.

T: Were you able to keep the stimulus control and competing response stuff together, and make use of them, in the evenings when things are often at their most difficult TTM-wise?

P: Not so much, no, and the pulling urges were really strong all week, too.

T: Sounds like it's been worse recently then – in the last few weeks before this one you'd been able to use the techniques and the pulling has been going down (shows the patient the graph of the previous weeks' pulling estimates) since we put the competing responses in place.

P: No, this week it's definitely up, although I didn't really do a good job with the monitoring so I'm not even sure how much worse it was.

T: Stronger urges, more pulling, less use of techniques, less hopefulness about your ability to do this work?

P: Yeah, all of that.

T: Well let's see if we can figure out together what's been contributing to that, OK?

P: OK. I actually thought you'd be mad at me, but you don't seem to be.

T: Well it's much more that I'm really sorry that you've had to go through such a tough week, and now we've got to put our heads together to figure it out. What did you make of it yourself as you thought about what's been going on?

P: Well remember when I told you in the beginning that I had some worries and fears that don't have much to do with hair pulling?

T: Sure – it sounded like you used to get really worried about germs, and about bad things happening to you if you didn't do your other rituals.

P: Yeah, those ones. Well they've been much worse in the last few weeks and I thought I could handle them, but they're kind of out of control now.

T: Did anything prompt their return, or did they just gradually increase over the last few weeks?

P: This is going to sound stupid, but I saw some commercials when I was watching TV a few weeks ago about a TV movie about bird flu hitting the U.S., and ever since it's been pretty hard with the worries about contamination and about having to wash a lot.

T: Avoiding stuff too?

P: Yeah, I'm really careful about where I put my hands, trying to stay out of places where I think the risk is higher, that kind of thing. I know it's not really likely, but I still can't stop thinking about it and when I think about it I can't help but wash, avoid, and try to protect myself and my family.

T: All of those things would be perfectly logical if the risk was high, and the OCD has got you thinking that this is one of those situations that it's better safe than sorry.

P: Exactly – even if it's probably not going to happen, what if it actually did? I can't get those pictures from the movie commercial out of my head, and now my OCD's got me adding my own face to some of them.

T: Sounds like it's been pretty tough on you.

P: And I got treated for this a long time ago and it's held up until now.

T: We know that the vulnerability to OCD remains even after good treatment, and sometimes stuff like this can just set it off.

P: Makes trich look pretty small in comparison right now.

T: Funny that you mention that – that's what I was thinking about too, and it raises some questions for us about how to proceed from here. The trich is worse in the last few weeks, but even so it sounds like the OCD is much bigger than that.

P: Yeah, it's gotten to the point where I even called out sick from work the last few days – I said I had a stomach virus, but that wasn't really true.

T: Did you call out because the OCD's got you wrapped up in general, or is there something specific about your work environment that OCD's saying is especially risky?

P: Definitely the latter – some of the people in my office have been traveling overseas recently, and I think they were in Istanbul at some point.

T: And the OCD is telling you that Istanbul is contaminated with bird flu?

P: Right – I heard on the news that there were some infected birds found there, and for me that means that the whole place is risky.

T: So going back in is going to be challenging.

P: More than that, I'm actually thinking about resigning.

T: What percentage of that decision has to do with OCD instead of job factors?

P: Probably 90%.

T: So the job's OK, but the contamination isn't?

P: Right.

T: That's a lot to have on your plate, and it confirms my suspicion that we might need to switch gears. I have some ideas about how to help with the OCD symptoms, but we'd need to agree to change our original plan of working on the trich.

P: I don't see how else we can do it – the pulling's bad right now, but it's nothing compared to the OCD at the moment.

T: And in all the time we've been working on the trich I never once heard you say that it's leading you to make big life decisions that might not be in your best interests, like quitting a job you generally like.

P: I think you're right – we should switch to the OCD.

T: Well let's think through now what that would look like, and what we're going to do about the trich in the meantime. Seems like we ought to keep some of the same things in place that were helping previously, but that we should really concentrate our efforts on reducing the OCD symptoms right now – after all, if we do that successfully, it might be the case that we indirectly work on the trich by reducing the exacerbating factors.

P: Makes sense – I'm willing to try to work on the OCD.

T: Good, then, now let me grab a measure of OCD symptoms so I can get a better sense of how bad things are OCD-wise at the moment . . .

CHAPTER 15

ATTENDING TO THE CONTEXT:
Module 5: Family-Based Approaches

Family issues often arise in the context of TTM treatment, and on occasion prove sufficiently prominent and interfering as to warrant additional clinical attention. This module is intended for use when family matters extend beyond what might generally be expected in the context of conducting psychotherapy for a specific disorder. Certainly those clinicians who treat youth are more likely to have to consider additional family-based treatment techniques and approaches, but even those who treat adults may need to include some family work when the family relationships are close and/or problematic. Accordingly, we will focus most of our attention on delivering family-based interventions when a child or adolescent is the patient being treated for TTM, but will also include some examples of how to manage commonly encountered family difficulties when treating adults.

INVOLVING THE FAMILY IN THE TREATMENT OF YOUTH: STANDARD OPERATING PROCEDURE

With respect to family involvement, we must first remind the reader that the definitive studies of whether TTM and functional outcomes are improved when families are specifically included in treatment have yet to be done in pediatric TTM. Interestingly, the studies that have been completed in anxious youth comparing family-based to individual CBT approaches have generally been equivocal, with some studies suggesting an advantage for family based approaches, some studies failing to find a statistically significant or clinically meaningful difference, and others still indicating that individual CBT was superior to family based CBT. In the absence of data to drive the decisions about family involvement for youth with TTM specifically, we have tended to conduct individual CBT with some family involvement, with sufficient protocol flexibility to allow for more or less parent involvement than this depending on developmental factors and the degree of family involvement in patterns that exacerbate TTM and associated difficulties. In most sessions with children and adolescents we tend to begin the session by meeting the patient in the waiting room, greet the parent(s), bring the child to the treatment room, conduct the session for approximately 40 minutes, then return to the waiting room, bring the parents back to the treatment room, and meet with the patient and the family together for another 10–15 minutes. During this shared time, we ask the patient to summarize for the parent what was covered in the session, explain the theoretical rationale for chosen procedures, describe the assigned homework for the coming week, and then check in with the parent to see if there are any specific questions or issues they wish to raise.

We prefer the aforementioned session structure because it underscores the central role that the child or adolescent must play in treatment, which is especially important since attempting to "work around" an unmotivated youngster is generally not a steady pathway to successful outcome. The presentation of the session summary and the rationale for treatment procedures allows the therapist to check on the conceptual understanding of the treatment; we believe that the likelihood that the child or adolescent will continue to use treatment procedures is predicated on understanding why they are being chosen. We also use this session structure to reinforce for parents that the treatment "belongs" to the child, with the parent in a supportive role. Homework can be discussed with parent and child together, questions addressed, and the preferred stance of the parents can be reinforced by the therapist. With very young children there might be a point system put in place as well in which the child can earn rewards for successful utilization of techniques; we emphasize when putting these procedures in place that parent and child should agree up front about what the rewards will be, develop a tracking method to ensure accurate and timely reinforcement, and we also make sure to be clear that points earned should not be rescinded. The emphasis is placed on utilization of techniques (e.g., using fiddle toys in high risk situations) rather than on pulling per se, since we anticipate that pulling will be reduced anyway with the successful implementation of techniques and this also gets the family away from the impression that the child is being treated punitively for engaging in pulling behavior.

In most cases the approach described above will prove sufficient, and the therapist will be able to establish a regular pattern to the session that reinforces the important role the child plays in helping themselves get better, draws upon parental support and concern, and provides a helpful context from which the battle against TTM is viewed as a collaborative endeavor. There are exceptions, of course, and when family problems are so prominent or serious that keeping the focus on TTM does not appear to be in the child's best interest, the considerations raised in the comorbidity module about when to try to handle the family problems within the context of TTM treatment or to shift the focus to the family difficulties may well apply. The most obvious example of a situation in which the shift in focus must be made is if physical or sexual abuse in the family is uncovered. Our own data suggest that child physical or sexual abuse in youth with TTM is not at all common (DeTore et al., 2006), but when present compliance with reporting laws and and ensuring the child's safety become the main priorities in treatment. Below we describe several other family-related situations that may warrant clinical attention as well; some of these problems might be solved without suspending focus on TTM, but the decision to do so will be made at least in part by the success of an initial attempt to deal with the family matter without shifting away from TTM for an extended period of time.

MISUNDERSTANDING WITHIN THE FAMILY ABOUT THE NATURE OF TTM

The psychoeducation that we provide routinely in the core TTM treatment package emphasizes the putative neurobiological nature of the disorder and emphasizes that TTM is nobody's fault, is maintained via reinforcement, and can be altered by improving awareness of pulling urges, blocking pulling via stimulus control methods, and reinforcing urges to pull in the context of habit reversal training by engaging in a competing response that is incompatible with pulling. On occasion, however, parents of youth with TTM may have their own hypotheses about why their child is pulling that do not converge with what is actually known about the disorder empirically and/or is inconsistent with developing the collaborative spirit that we believe is critical to successful treatment. For example, we have encountered parents who have emphasized their view that the child is pulling because they know how difficult pulling is on the parents. Our advice in this situation is to take the opportunity to acknowledge that TTM affects everyone in the family, to explore the interactional patterns between family conflict and pulling behavior to see if any clear patterns emerge, and to bring the parents and the child back to the conceptual model of TTM to demonstrate how negative interactions about pulling such as blaming the child for the parents' suffering is unlikely to reduce pulling but instead is likely to increase stress, which then feeds back in our model to increase urges to pull. We take this approach to help get parents and patients to get out of the "blame game" where each tries to convince the other that their suffering is greater, but without a constructive end in sight. When such patterns emerge, we also encourage therapists to check in with the child to determine whether the psychoeducation about TTM has reduced this tendency or had no effect – if the latter, perhaps some individual time with the parents reiterating the likely effect of this criticism and problem solving about how to manage their own feelings about their child's TTM may be warranted.

Another common misconception that can negatively impact treatment is when the parents become very focused on identifying the precise cause of TTM; this might be even more complicated if the parents are convinced that something they did or something their partner did led to the development of TTM. We have spoken to many parents who have recalled with much affect how they handled the earliest signs of TTM in their child (e.g., stroking and twirling hair), and have wondered whether a reaction they perceive as harsh or unaccepting led to the perpetuation of the hairpulling. Again we come back to the conceptual model, which highlights the fact that there is no single or necessary input that must occur in order for TTM to begin, and we also point out that our model does not contain a specific box for "suboptimal parental response to initial pulling episodes," suggesting that we as experts in this area do not believe that this is a likely catalyst for pulling. For parents who have other theories about why TTM began and focus on those events or reactions (e.g., hospitalization of a child at a young age, negative first sleepover camp experiences for the child), we emphasize that the treatment approach we espouse does not require us to identify a definitive precipitating event, but instead focuses on the maintenance of current pulling rather than exploration of the context for its onset. Here we draw on the treatment outcome literature, which does not include any randomized studies suggesting that identification of etiological factors in and of themselves is associated with excellent acute outcome and maintenance of gains.

Perhaps by virtue of working in clinics that are known for OCD treatment, we have also occasionally met with parents whose own working models of TTM heavily emphasizes the central role of "obsessions" that the parents believe are necessarily present and driving pulling. These parents can sometimes become frustrated with the child's repeated insistence that he or she was not thinking about anything in particular when the pulling began – parents with this more cognition-driven model sometimes interpret this response from the child as unwillingness to "be honest" or intentionally withholding information from the parent and the therapist that is likely to be helpful in reducing pulling. Here again our initial attempt to address this problem is to return to the conceptual model, to discuss the fact that many if not most TTM patients cannot identify a thought that precipitates pulling, and reiterate that TTM is not viewed as an especially "cognitive" disorder. We attempt to use this opportunity to emphasize that improving awareness may therefore play a critical role in treatment given that the typical TTM patient may not have a cognitive "warning sign" that pulling urges are about to intensify. With this and with all of the misunderstandings we mentioned above, we wish to remind therapists that an empathic rather than a judgmental tone in trying to correct these misunderstandings is always going to be best, regardless of whether the intervention corrects the misunderstanding. Put another way, John March's adage that "kindness is always better than yelling" applies to the families being seen as well as the therapists who see them.

Parents of children and adolescents with TTM are not the only people whose misconceptions about the nature of TTM might inadvertently derail standard TTM treatment. In our work with adults we have encountered spouses and partners whose beliefs about TTM can interfere with delivery of standard treatment and hence might be a target for remediation as well. "She's doing this because she hates herself," "He pulls at night in the bathroom in order to avoid being with me," and other such theories can be a source of relationship tension and unhappiness that can, as the conceptual model highlights, thereby indirectly strengthen urges to pull. Although we do not routinely involve spouses, partners, friends, adult children, or other key figures in treatment, when we hear from our patients that the theories and reactions of loved ones are proving to be harmful rather than helpful, with the patient's agreement we will invite the relevant party to a treatment session to discuss the nature of TTM, present the conceptual model, demonstrate how the treatment procedures flow from our theoretical model, and offer to answer any questions or concerns. These sessions are often of considerable value, both in improving understanding about TTM and its treatment but also allowing the patient and the relevant person in their life an opportunity to discuss TTM openly in the presence of a knowledgeable professional. When the problems persist beyond these meetings, we also may spend subsequent session time role-playing with a patient how to respond when advice or comments from a well meaning but misguided family member is provided without solicitation by the patient.

PARENTAL OVERINVOLVEMENT AND PREOCCUPATION WITH TTM

Watching as your child suffers is extremely difficult for most parents and, in the case of parents of children with TTM, recognizing that the suffering takes place as a result of the child's own behavior makes this difficult task all the more complicated. Many parents are therefore highly motivated to help their children with TTM to find proper treatment, and sometimes this extends to implementing the treatment as well. Parental interest and involvement in treatment is likely to be central to its success, and we do not wish to convey that youth with TTM should be treated without taking this central context into account. Nevertheless, there are clinical situations in which parental involvement hinders treatment progress and results in increased urges to pull. This might become obvious early on in treatment when parents break down in front of the child when discussing how terrible the child's TTM make the parent feel, or when questions posed to the child by the therapists are routinely answered by the parent or when the child's answers are routinely contradicted by the parent (e.g., "No it's not at all like that – you do pull frequently when you're doing your homework"). To an extent the information provided by a second set of eyes can be invaluable, especially when considering the fact that pulling often begins outside of awareness. On the other hand, when the parent's adamant tone suggests that they have taken a stance whereby they must "report the truth" or "tell on" the child to the therapist, some subtle attempts to remediate the potential problem should be attempted. For example, a therapist might say to such a parent, "I think it's going to be helpful at this early stage of treatment to provide us with information about what you're seeing with the child's pulling, since of course pulling often starts before the person is even aware of it, almost like the hand has a mind of its own. Now let's see how (Child's name) would like that information conveyed so they can make the most use of it – would you prefer that Mom or Dad tell you right away, or that they tell you later on when you're working on your monitoring homework?" This stance reinforces that the desire to provide such information is natural and expected, but that the timing and the way the information is conveyed is of importance as well. Once this initial intervention is attempted, the therapist should examine the monitoring forms and inquire directly of the child as to whether the parent(s) has been able or unable to follow the guidelines for conveying information about pulling to the child during the week. If there has not been good follow-through, here again it might be useful to bring the parent in for some time with the therapist and the patient together to feed this information back to the parent and problem solve around how best to minimize the provision of information about pulling in ways and at times when it is not likely to be fully grasped or appreciated.

When these attempts still do not slow down the tendency of the parent to become the "Trich Police," the therapist must increase their attention to the potentially damaging effects of this approach on the child's willingness to work on the pulling. In certain cases, perhaps the most persistent ones or the most interpersonally problematic ones, this conversation might be best attempted with the parent alone and proceed as follows: "I know that we all have the same goal in mind, which is to help your child better understand and more successfully battle with her very intense urges to pull, and your enthusiasm for achieving that goal that is much appreciated. On the other hand, I'm really concerned that your pointing out immediately to your child each and every time her hand goes to her head in your presence might not be having the effect that we'd prefer, which is to improve awareness without substantially increasing interpersonal tension and stress. We know that for many people this kind of stress can actually increase urges to pull, so we need to find a more effective way for you to share your observations about your daughter's pulling without inadvertently making the job more difficult. Let's take some time to go over how to do that – we can really benefit from what you're seeing, but at the same time it's likely that this information would be more useful to your daughter if it was conveyed differently or at a different time, say later, when she's not pulling actively."

Parents often take the child's pulling very seriously, and accordingly TTM and the attempts to combat it can become a dominant theme at the dinner table each night. Some children do not mind this focus, but most might find it embarrassing, shame-producing, and isolating, especially when these discussions take place in the presence of siblings who do not happen to have the disorder. We encourage parents to be mindful of the potential untoward effects of discussing TTM at great lengths in such contexts, or to elaborate upon TTM and its treatment in the child's presences with extended family, neighbors, and friends. One family we treated responded to our feedback about this kind of process by creating a "Trich Pow-wow" time after completion of school homework but before preparation for bed. The Trich Pow-wow was conducted in the child's room, by either mother or father depending on the night of the week, and was a private conversation in which the parent could review the monitoring sheet with the child, reward compliance with TTM homework tasks and with monitoring, and could share privately with the child his or her observations about the child's pulling throughout the day. They would write up a "Recommendations" list each night consisting of one or two key points, and this would be kept with the monitoring sheets to be shared with the therapists but, perhaps most importantly, as grist for the next night's "Pow-wow." This tradition was eventually faded to a weekly meeting once the child and the parent were confident that the child was able to take responsibility for the treatment, and it grew more informal from there as the child was able to successfully implement the treatment procedures being taught. We encourage this kind of creativity within the family that would satisfy the parent's need to be helpful and involved while respecting and encouraging the child's sense of autonomy and control, although we also recognize that there are some cases where the parent's issues would preclude such a smooth transition to a lesser role. In those cases we might empathize with the parent about how difficult it is to let go but at the same time reiterate the importance of doing so for the child's long-term outcomes with TTM and more broadly.

PARENTAL IMPATIENCE WITH THE PACE OF TREATMENT

Another problem we have encountered on occasion in our work with TTM and families involves parental impatience with the pace of treatment. We emphasize up front that TTM is a complex habit with underlying neurobiological correlates, and hence we do not expect Rome to be built in a day in reducing the pulling and the associated urges to pull. To reinforce this notion we ask parents about whether they have ever quit smoking, engaged in a weight loss program, or overcome other kinds of problem behaviors. We ask them to recall from their own experiences whether the behavior was reduced immediately, whether there was a lag between cutting back on the behavior itself and dissipation of urges to do so, and whether the task was difficult or not. Often times this conversation allows us a foot in the door for promoting patience with the child's attempts to reduce the pulling behavior, and we refer back to that conversation if we sense in our time with the parents that they expect faster progress than is realistically possible. We also convey to the family that our protocol is designed to take 3–4 months to implement specifically because we expect it will take that long to get all of the pieces in place and implemented regularly, and if we thought we could do so much faster we would have designed the treatment differently for the sake of efficiency. Parents can get frustrated if they see that a child is still pulling after several weeks, and we reinforce the idea that we can use these data to help us better understand which elements of the protocol need to be shored up or augmented with other procedures. We point out that the data from treatment outcome studies in adults and children suggest that it is likely that pulling urges and even some pulling behavior is likely to persist, and thus we should adopt from the start a long-term view of how to put all of the relevant aspects of the protocol in place. We also underscore that elimination of pulling or at least substantial reduction of pulling is an important goal of treatment but not the only goal: helping the child to understand the disorder better, feel less to blame for it, learn how it works for them, learn which techniques are most effective for them, and accept themselves more fully as human beings regardless of the status of the pulling are each important goals as well, and that achievement of these goals might enhance pulling outcomes either immediately or down the road when the child feels more ready to work on the pulling per se.

Parents may also get confused about why the context shift can have such a strong influence over the pulling behavior and even the urges to pull. For example, parents might see that the child is able to reduce and even eliminate pulling in front of other people at school yet persists in pulling at home when alone in her room. This can lead to feelings that the child "isn't trying," which in turn can increase parental vigilance and pressure, which presumably will work against achieving the goal of pulling and urge reduction. In discussing these issues, we return to the conceptual model to demonstrate how environmental cues might either suppress or exacerbate pulling behaviors, and that what we learned about how the child was able to corral pulling at school might prove extremely useful in combating urges at home: for example, the child might be less likely to begin pulling when other people are present out of concern for what others might think if they saw the child engaging in pulling, and thus studying in her room alone might be temporarily replaced by studying in the living room where it is at least possible for other family members to enter unannounced. We suggest to parents that treating TTM is much like apple picking in that you grab the low-lying fruit first, then work your way up to the more difficult to reach areas. By using this analogy we underscore that we believe that having easier and harder places in which to stop pulling is inherent, is expected, and does not necessarily suggest lack of motivation on the child's part.

FAILURE TO REINFORCE EFFORT

With young children especially but perhaps even across the developmental spectrum, one of the most reinforcing aspects of working on reducing pulling is the positive attention that one receives for taking on a difficult job and trying to do your best. For the very young children we augment social reinforcement with other rewards for complying with treatment, completing homework assignments, etc., because we recognize that young children may not be sufficiently motivated by an abstract goal of reducing pulling urges and the impact of TTM on their lives years down the road. It is therefore critical that if a point system is put into place that parents and therapists alike take the implementation of this system according to the previously agreed parameters very seriously, and stick to the agreements about reviewing the successes, providing social and other more tangible reinforcement as discussed, and refrain from reworking the system without extensive discussion and agreement. Often failure to provide reinforcement is a function of how busy life can be for parent and child – we have occasionally asked patients to let us know how the reward systems are working only to be told "we forgot to do it." These problems can usually be remediated relatively easily via problem solving: placing the chart in a place where it serves as a reminder to the parent and the child to review and update it, setting up a special time each night to discuss the program and implement the rewards, and reiterating to the parent and the child how the reward system can help make difficult tasks more easy. We then encourage therapists to check in routinely to make sure that initial and seemingly benign problems with follow-through are reduced – regularly devoting some session time to the reward system is a good way to improve compliance and to model for the family how organizing the time to review the homework can be worked in regularly to discussions about TTM more broadly.

Sometimes the failure to reinforce effort is not simply a function of mutual busyness, but rather the result of parental misgivings about "bribery." Those of us who work with families often encounter this initial reluctance, and our responses often come from the power of reinforcement in the functioning of adults and can be conveyed in a somewhat humorous tone: "Though I really like my job and think that the things I do here are important both for me and for the people that I work with, I also think that if University officials were to withdraw their reinforcement for my efforts – meaning stop making those monthly direct deposits into my bank account – I would likely not like my job as much over time, and eventually would stop doing it." We encourage parents to think about this aspect of the treatment as fundamentally important to priming the motivational pump, and we also tell parents that as the treatment and its results become reinforcing, the external reinforcers can eventually be faded. Parents also on occasion withhold or rescind earned reinforcers because of unrelated transgressions, such as the child talking back to the parents, getting a bad grade at school, or fighting with a sibling. In such cases we try to get parents to see the potential for this kind of breach to undermine the motivation of the child to do the work necessary to reduce pulling, and to honor the agreement about reinforcing efforts to work the program regardless of what else was going on in terms of discipline. The reward system should be treated as immutable unless changes are agreed upon up front, and other TTM-irrelevant disciplinary issues should be addressed separately. We remind parents that we do not expect them to give the child a "free pass" for transgressions simply because they are in treatment for TTM, but rather to think about the TTM reward system and the other issues as separate matters entirely.

DISAGREEMENTS AND PROBLEMS UNRELATED TO TTM

We have also encountered times when family arguments and disagreements about other matters become so prominent that a shift to address these issues becomes important. For example, disagreements about school problems can emerge in children with TTM that must take precedence over treating the pulling; sometimes these problems are related to TTM (e.g., patient cannot study effectively because studying prompts urges to pull, and pulling interferes with the child's concentration) and sometimes they are unrelated (e.g., child fails to hand in schoolwork on time because of a general pattern of procrastination). The first step in these circumstances it to try to parse out the effects of TTM on the observed academic problem, to explore the effect of the problem on pulling urges regardless of whether the problem itself was TTM-related, and to develop a plan of action to address the academic difficulty. When the problem is an acute one and likely to be addressed rather easily, this can often be accomplished without shifting the treatment away from pulling, but rather by devoting some session time to solving the problem and then exploring with the child and the family the effects of such problems on pulling as a chance to learn more about the presentation of TTM in this particular child. There are occasions when school personnel, tutors, and other professionals from the education field may be needed to help sort out the academic difficulties that the student is encountering; our own data suggest that attentional and learning problems might occur in children and adolescents with TTM at higher rates than what might be expected by chance (Tolin et al., 2006), so it is important to help the family recognize the importance of garnering academic resources that might be needed.

Family squabbles and disagreements may also emerge about a host of other content areas, and it is important to determine whether these are new or repeated problems, to determine how the family tends to go about solving such disagreements, and to judge whether the problem is sufficiently impairing as to preclude continuing to take a focused approach to TTM. As we discussed in the chapter on comorbidity, we wish to lay out the choices as follows: 1) remain focused on TTM and devote limited session time to the family problem; 2) turn to address the family problem and temporarily suspend focus on TTM, but with an intent to return to TTM treatment soon; 3) suspend TTM treatment indefinitely and devote session time to dealing with the emergent family problems; or 4) refer for family counseling, and invite the family to resume TTM treatment when the family crisis or problems are under better control. The severity of the problem, expertise of the therapist, motivation of the child and family to focus on one problem or the other, and other such factors will influence this decision, but we encourage therapists to monitor the situation to ensure that the focus selected is truly the one in the best interest of the client, which in the context we have described would be the child. We have had similar situations emerge with our adult patients as well, however: one woman who came for TTM treatment and identified marital stress as contributing to her urges to pull reported that her husband had let her know that he was seriously considering a divorce, that the decision had little if anything to do with her pulling, and that he would like to try to work on the marriage before taking legal action. We inquired about the patient's goals in light of this discussion, and when she made it clear that she too would like to work on the relationship then we made a clinical referral and suspended the TTM treatment indefinitely. Years later this patient, by then divorced, returned to work on the TTM which, she noted, had worsened in the wake of the break-up, reduced somewhat after getting her life back together, and had begun to increase again after having accepted a promotion at work that was associated with increased responsibility and stress.

CHAPTER 16

GETTING SUPPORT:

Module 6: Group Therapy and Other Methods to Improve Access to Care

To this point, all of the procedures in this book have been described from a standpoint of individual therapy. However, in clinical practice much treatment is provided in groups, rather than in an individual format. Two primary factors stand out as reasons to consider group, rather than individual, therapy:

- Group therapy is cost-effective. In this era of managed health care, many clinicians are under pressure to come up with the most cost-effective treatment option. In general, CBT compares quite favorably with medications in terms of cost-effectiveness. For example, research with anxiety-disordered patients (Otto, Pollack, & Maki, 2000) has shown that CBT and medications were roughly cost-equivalent during the acute phase of treatment. The cost of treatments differed, however, after acute treatment, because CBT typically is not continued as long as medications. One year after treatment, the cost of individual CBT was only 59% of the cost of medications, with cost-effectiveness ratios (the cost of treatment divided by the degree of clinical improvement) showing an identical pattern. Furthermore, group CBT was even less expensive, and more cost-effective, than individual CBT. Treating multiple patients at the same time invariably contains health care costs.
- Group therapy contains a social component that may not be present in individual therapy. We have heard countless patients tell us that, before coming to treatment, they thought they were the only ones in the world who suffered from

this problem (many of them were not even aware that the problem had a name!). As a result, many people enter group therapy with an initial sense of apprehension, embarrassment, or shame. However, when they see others with noticeable alopecia, and hear others' stories about pulling and their unsuccessful attempts to stop, these patients typically experience relief that they are not alone. Yalom (1995) refers to this concept as "universality" (p. 5). The group setting also provides a nice venue for patients to exchange ideas about how to stop pulling, and to discuss what has and has not worked for them.

Group therapy generally appears to be an efficacious means of delivering CBT, although results comparing group to individual CBT are mixed. One study of group vs. individual therapy for OCD, for example (Fals-Stewart, Marks, & Schafer, 1993), found that both treatment conditions resulted in similar decreases in symptom severity, and both were superior to a relaxation-only condition; similar outcomes were found recently in Australia for individual versus group approaches in treating OCD in children and adolescents (Barrett et al., 2004). In both studies, gains from group treatment were maintained over a 6-month follow-up period. Profile analysis in the Fals-Stewart et al. (1993) study indicated that patients receiving individual CBT responded to treatment more rapidly than did those receiving group CBT. Similar findings have been reported for CBT with substance-abusing adults, with both treatment modalities showing equivalent results (Marques & Formigoni, 2001). Anxious children appear to respond equally well to group CBT as to individual treatment, although very socially anxious children may respond more favorably to individual CBT (Manassis et al., 2002). In a study of obese adults (Renjilian et al., 2001), patients appeared to respond better to group CBT than to individual CBT, regardless of whether they expressed an initial preference for group or individual treatment. Other studies have found group CBT to be less efficacious than individual CBT for social phobia (Stangier, Heidenreich, Peitz, Lauterbach, & Clark, 2003), although previous research had demonstrated the opposite (Scholing & Emmelkamp, 1993). Individual CBT appears superior to group CBT in the treatment of bulimia nervosa (Chen et al., 2003). Individual CBT was more effective than a supportive group intervention for depressed, medically compromised patients (Mohr, Boudewyn, Goodkin, Bostrom, & Epstein, 2001), although the difference in outcomes could be attributable to differences in treatment modality (CBT vs. supportive therapy), rather than the individual vs. group format.

To date, there have been very few investigations of the use of group interventions to treat TTM. Stanley and Mouton (1996) modified habit reversal training for a group format; an initial study of three patients found that all three showed marked reductions in time spent pulling, number of hairs pulled, and overall TTM severity. In a subsequent study, the intervention was effective for four out of five group patients at post-treatment; however, at 6-month follow-up, only two out of the five continued to show clinically significant reductions in hair pulling (Mouton & Stanley, 1996). Although this is a relatively poor long-term outcome, this does not necessarily point to a shortcoming of the use of groups; similarly high relapse rates have been documented in individual CBT (Lerner et al., 1998).

Recently, Diefenbach et al. (2006) compared a more comprehensive form of group CBT to supportive group therapy for adult patients with TTM. After an initial baseline period during which no change in TTM symptoms was noted, 24 adult TTM patients were randomly assigned to either a CBT group ($n = 12$) or a supportive group ($n = 12$). Number of patients in each group ranged from 3–6. The groups each met for 8 weekly sessions, with each session lasting 1.5 hours. The CBT groups received psychoeducation (see Chapter 2), awareness training (see Chapter 7), stimulus control (see Chapter 8), competing response training (see Chapter 9), relaxation training (see Chapter 12), cognitive restructuring (see Chapter 13), and relapse prevention (see Chapter 10). Each session was followed by homework assignments to be practiced during the week. The supportive therapy groups received a nondirective, supportive series of discussions. During these discussions, patients were free to discuss TTM, but the therapist provided no specific strategies for reducing hair pulling. Group CBT resulted in significant decreases in hair pulling symptoms at post-treatment, whereas supportive therapy did not. Ratings of hair loss by evaluators who were blind to treatment condition suggested that CBT patients had less alopecia at post-treatment and at 1- and 3-month follow-ups than did the supportive group patients. At post-treatment, 89% of the CBT group patients, compared to 30% of the supportive group patients, were rated "much improved" or "very much improved" on the Clinical Global Impressions (CGI) scale (Guy, 1976). By one-month follow-up, however, the CBT group showed some signs of relapse, with 57% of patients rated as "much improved" or "very much improved" on the CGI, compared to 30% of the supportive group patients. At three-month follow-up, the percentage of patients in each group receiving this rating was 50%. Thus, group CBT appears superior to supportive group therapy in the short term; however, as is the case in individual therapy (e.g., Lerner et al., 1998), it appears that more attention needs to be paid to issues of maintenance and relapse prevention (see Chapter 10). It may be that 8 sessions of group CBT was simply not sufficient for many patients to find long-term relief from hair pulling. Researchers and clinicians may wish to consider longer-term groups, or periodic "booster" group sessions.

Yalom (1995) has written extensively about the process of group psychotherapy. Primarily, he writes from the perspective of process-oriented existential and psychodynamic therapy; however, many of the principles he explicates apply equally well to CBT groups. His concept of universality has been mentioned above. Another particularly applicable aspect of successful group therapy is that of *cohesiveness*, or the attraction of each individual to the group itself. To the extent that each member of the group, whether process- or CBT-oriented, feels like they are a part of the group, and experience a sense of understanding, warmth, and respect from the other group members, the group might be said to possess a high degree of cohesiveness. The importance of group cohesiveness in CBT has not been studied formally to our knowledge; however, our experience suggests that it is a critical factor in treatment process and outcome. Groups that rely on an exclusively didactic style, with the therapist providing "lectures" to the group, do not seem to be particularly effective. In many respects, this parallels the process of individual therapy: simply telling the patient about the model of TTM and walking them through the steps of competing response training, stimulus control, etc., tends to elicit passivity, resistance, non-adherence, or premature treatment discontinuation. In individual therapy, the techniques of CBT are most effective when they are delivered within the context of a warm, understanding, and respectful therapeutic relationship, with an emphasis on collaboration and back-and-forth discussion. So it is, too, with group therapy; however, group therapy raises the additional issue of requiring these relationship factors not only with the therapist, but also with the other group members.

To facilitate group cohesiveness, our preference is to limit didactic presentations to only a portion of each group session. Certainly, the therapist has some information that must be passed along to the group members in order for treatment to be effective; it is unlikely, for example, that competing response strategies will spontaneously "pop up" during a nondirective group discussion. However, we also take care to spend time in each group allowing each patient to talk. In some sessions, particularly early ones, patients may wish to spend most of the time talking about hair pulling. However, in other sessions, patients may have other things on their minds, such as pressures at school or work, family concerns, even current events. We see these topics as valid and valuable, even though they may not technically fit with the therapy modules in this book, or may deviate from the therapist's agenda for the session. The therapist who attempts to force his/her agenda against the wishes of the group is asking for trouble. Rather, as these other issues come up, we use them as a way to facilitate group cohesion by asking questions such as, "Has anyone else ever felt this way?" or "Bob, what do you think about what Susan just said?"

That said, without some kind of agenda for group meetings, the group is likely to devolve into a nondirective "rap group," which, although perhaps personally satisfying, is unlikely to result in substantial behavior change. Therefore, we usually begin each group with a brief statement (or writing on a blackboard) about our agenda for the group, as well as its rationale; for example, "What I have in mind for today is to teach you a strategy called competing response training. This is an exercise that's designed to help you resist the urge to pull, and it has helped a lot of people cut down on their pulling. Before we get to that, though, I'd like to hear about how things have been going for you, and what's been on your mind. Who would like to start?" In this manner, the therapist has identified a goal for the day, and provided a reason for introducing that topic. However, he/she also is not monopolizing group time, and provides a venue for group members to speak.

Another potential advantage of group approaches for TTM is that they help spread out the already thin resources for TTM treatment that exist in most U.S. states and countries. A recent finding from the Trichotillomania Impact Study highlighted the importance of doing so: only 15% of respondents to the TIP who reported having sought treatment for TTM described their treatment provider as a "TTM expert" or "very knowledgeable" about TTM (Woods et al., 2006). Group treatments would allow multiple patients to be seen at one time, thus shortening waitlists and establishing an ongoing system of support even after group treatment has completed.

Recently in TTM another approach to improving access to care has been attempted, a web-based, interactive, self-help program called StopPulling.com (Mouton-Odum et al., 2006). This program might be especially important in areas of the country and the world where TTM expertise cannot be found within a reasonable distance which, sadly enough, still describes most regions nationally and internationally. The program presents modules in Assessment, Intervention, and Maintenance in accordance with a cognitive-behaviorally oriented approach. Data collected from 265 program users during the first year of public availability of the program indicated that users' TTM symptoms were reduced from pre- to post-use, with evidence for a positive relationship between length of use in sessions and degree of TTM symptom reduction.

StopPulling.com may also prove useful for individuals who, even though they are fortunate enough to have local TTM expertise, are simply not ready to present for treatment in person. Similarly, self-help books may also play an important role in improving access to care in TTM and in providing individuals who feel they are not ready for or cannot afford face-to-face contact, and there are a number of excellent volumes already published for adults (e.g., Keuthen et al., 2001; Penzel, 2003) and for children and adolescents (e.g., Golomb & Vavrichek, 1999). It is our hope that this manual, by providing a comprehensive CBT approach to TTM, will also assist with the important goal of improving access to care for TTM sufferers.

PART 4

RESOURCES FOR CLINICIANS, PATIENTS, AND FAMILIES

LIST OF PROFESSIONAL AND INFORMATIONAL SOURCES FOR CLINICIANS, PATIENTS AND FAMILIES

TTM-SPECIFIC RESOURCES

TRICHOTILLOMANIA LEARNING CENTER

http://www.trich.org/index.asp
The Trichotillomania Learning Center (TLC) is a non-profit resource for individuals who pull hair or pick their skin, and also for their families and friends, medical and mental health professionals, and others interested in learning about these often-misunderstood problems. TLC staff is available to answer questions, provide professional referrals, or just listen – at 831–457–1004.

OTHER RESOURCES

OC FOUNDATION

http://www.ocfoundation.org/
The Obsessive-Compulsive Foundation (OCF) is an international not-for-profit organization composed of people with obsessive compulsive disorder (OCD) and related disorders, their families, friends, professionals and other concerned individuals.

Anxiety Disorders Association of America

http://www.adaa.org/

The Anxiety Disorders Association of America (ADAA) is a nonprofit organization whose mission is to promote the prevention, treatment and cure of anxiety disorders and to improve the lives of all people who suffer from them.

TTM-SPECIFIC SELF-HELP BOOKS

Golomb, R. G., Vavrichek, S. M. (1999). *The hair pulling "habit" and you: how to solve the trichotillomania puzzle (rev ed).* Silver Spring, MD: Writer's Cooperative of Greater Washington. Book for children and teenagers.

Keuthen, N. J., Stein,D. J., Christenson, G. A. (2001). *Help for hair pullers: Understanding and coping with trichotillomania.* Oakland, CA, US: New Harbinger.

Book for adults.

Penzel, F. (2003). The hair-pulling problem: A complete guide to trichotillomania. New York: Oxford University Press.

Book for adults with a chapter on TTM and your child.

FUNCTIONAL ASSESSMENT
OF TRICHOTILLOMANIA

Name _____   **Date** _____

Pulling sites (check all that apply)

☐ Scalp   ☐ Pubic region
☐ Eyebrows   ☐ Face
☐ Eyelashes   ☐ Arms
☐ Armpits   ☐ Legs
☐ Chest   ☐ Other _____

List primary pulling sites, in order:

	Pulling Site	How many times per typical day?	How many hairs pulled per typical session?
1.			
2.			
3.			

Other body-focused repetitive behaviors:

☐ Skin picking   ☐ Nose picking
☐ Nail biting or picking   ☐ Hair twirling or rubbing
☐ Knuckle cracking   ☐ Tics (specify) _____
☐ Thumb or finger sucking   ☐ Other _____
☐ Tongue, lip, or cheek biting

Pulling Triggers

Settings (list in order of most common)

Setting (e.g., bedroom)	Other variables that mediate this setting (e.g., presence or absence of others)	What percentage of pulling occurs in this setting?
1.		
2.		
3.		

Activities (list in order of most common)

Activity (e.g., watching TV)	Other variables that mediate this activity (e.g., presence or absence of others)	What percentage of pulling occurs during this activity?
1.		
2.		
3.		

Postural triggers (list in order of most common)

Posture (e.g., lying down)	Other variables that mediate this setting (e.g., hands behind head or at sides)	What percentage of pulling occurs in this posture?
1.		
2.		
3.		

Triggering thoughts (list in order of most common)

Thought (e.g., "I have too much to do today")	Other variables that mediate this setting (e.g., falling behind in tasks)	What percentage of pulling occurs after this thought?
1.		
2.		
3.		

Triggering emotions (list in order of most common)

Emotion (e.g., anxiety)	Other variables that mediate this setting (e.g., availability of medications)	What percentage of pulling occurs after feeling this way?
1.		
2.		
3.		

Triggering physiological sensations (list in order of most common)

Sensation (e.g., muscle tension)	Other variables that mediate this setting (e.g., availability of medications)	What percentage of pulling occurs after feeling this way?
1.		
2.		
3.		

Triggering arousal level

☐ Hyperarousal (e.g., hyper, tense, scattered)   ☐ Hypoarousal (e.g., bored, tired, sleepy)

Presence of urges to pull

☐ Yes (describe) _____ ☐ No

Pre-Pulling Events

Preparatory "grooming"-like behaviors (e.g., touching hair or face)

☐ Yes (describe) _____ ☐ No

Tactile or visual cues

☐ Yes (describe) _____ ☐ No

Change in thoughts, feelings, or physiological sensations

☐ Yes (describe) _____ ☐ No

Urges to pull

☐ Yes (describe) _____ ☐ No

Pulling Behaviors and Post-Pulling Events

Detailed description of the pulling behavior:

Changes in thoughts, feelings, or physiological sensations during and immediately after pulling:

☐ Increased pain   ☐ Decreased boredom
☐ Increased pleasure   ☐ Satisfaction
☐ Decreased anxiety/tension   ☐ Distraction from unpleasant thoughts
☐ Decreased sadness   ☐ Other _____
☐ Decreased anger

Visual behaviors with the pulled hair:

☐ Looks at hair   ☐ Looks for root
☐ Inspects color of root   ☐ Other _____

Tactile behaviors with the pulled hair:

☐ Rolls hair between fingers   ☐ Touches, squeezes, or bursts root
☐ Breaks hair   ☐ Weaves hair between fingers
☐ Sticks root to something   ☐ Other _____

Oral behaviors with the pulled hair:

☐ Rubs hair on lips   ☐ Passes hair between lips
☐ Puts hair in mouth   ☐ Bites root
☐ Swallows hair*   ☐ Other _____

*Note: excessive trichophagia may be associated with gastrointestinal complications. Inquire about gastrointestinal problems (e.g., upset stomach, constipation) and consider a medical referral if needed.

Method of discarding the pulled hair:

Changes in thoughts, feelings, or physiological sensations after the post-pulling behaviors:

☐ Decreased pulling-related pain   ☐ Decreased boredom
☐ Increased pleasure   ☐ Satisfaction
☐ Decreased anxiety/tension   ☐ Distraction from unpleasant thoughts
☐ Decreased sadness   ☐ Other _____
☐ Decreased anger

Delayed consequences of pulling:

☐   Grooming-related consequences   Describe

☐   Physical health consequences   Describe

☐   Social interaction consequences   Describe

☐   Recreational consequences   Describe

☐   Work and productivity consequences   Describe

☐   Emotional consequences   Describe

Hair-Pulling Diagram for (Name) _____

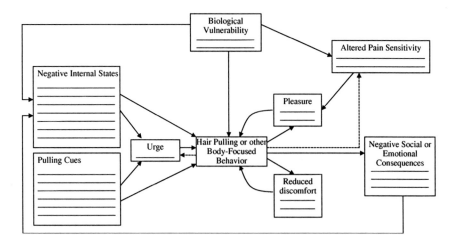

REFERENCES

Abrams, D. B., & Wilson, G. T. (1979). Self-monitoring and reactivity in the modification of cigarette smoking. *Journal of Consulting and Clinical Psychology, 47*, 243–251.

Adam, B. S., & Kashani, J. H. (1990). Trichotillomania in children and adolescents: review of the literature and case report. *Child Psychiatry and Human Development, 20*, 159–168.

Agras, W. S., Southam, M. A., & Taylor, C. B. (1983). Long-term persistence of relaxation-induced blood pressure lowering during the working day. *Journal of Consulting and Clinical Psychology, 51*, 792–794.

Ambrosini, P. J. (2000). Historical development and present status of the schedule for affective disorders and schizophrenia for school-age children (K-SADS). *Journal of the American Academy of Child and Adolescent Psychiatry, 39*, 49–58.

American Psychiatric Association. (1987). *Diagnostic and statistical manual of mental disorders* (3rd Revised ed.). Washington, DC: Author.

American Psychiatric Association. (2000). *Diagnostic and statistical manual of mental disorders (4th Edition-Text Revision)*. Washington, DC: Author.

Antony, M. M., Bieling, P. J., Cox, B. J., Enns, M. W., & Swinson, R. P. (1998). Psychometric properties of the 42-item and 21-item versions of the Depression Anxiety Stress Scales (DASS) in clinical groups and a community sample. *Psychological Assessment, 10*, 176–181.

Azrin, N. H., Kaplan, S. J., & Foxx, R. M. (1973). Autism reversal: eliminating stereotyped self-stimulation of retarded individuals. *Am J Ment Defic, 78*, 241–248.

Azrin, N. H., & Nunn, R. G. (1973). Habit-reversal: A method of eliminating nervous habits and tics. *Behaviour Research and Therapy, 11*, 619–628.

Azrin, N. H., Nunn, R. G., & Frantz, S. E. (1980). Treatment of hair pulling (trichotillomania): A comparative study of habit reversal and negative practice training. *Journal of Behavior Therapy and Experimental Psychiatry, 11*, 13–20.

Azrin, N. H., Nunn, R. G., & Frantz-Renshaw, S. E. (1982). Habit reversal vs negative practice treatment of self-destructive oral habits (biting, chewing or licking of the lips, cheeks, tongue or palate). *Journal of Behavior Therapy and Experimental Psychiatry, 13*, 49–54.

Barlow, D. H., & Hersen, M. (1984). *Single case experimental designs: Strategies for studying behavior change*. New York: Pergamon Press.

Barrett, P., Healy-Farrell, L., & March, J. S. (2004). Cognitive-behavioral family treatment of childhood obsessive-compulsive disorder: A controlled trial. *Journal of the American Academy of Child & Adolescent Psychiatry, 43*, 46–62.

Barrett, R. P., & Shapiro, E. S. (1980). Treatment of stereotyped hair-pulling with overcorrection: A case study with long-term follow-up. *Journal of Behavior Therapy & Experimental Psychiatry, 11*, 317–320.

Begotka, A. M., Woods, D. W., & Wetterneck, C. T. (2003). The relationship between experiential avoidance and the severity of trichotillomania in a nonreferred sample. *Journal of Behavior Therapy and Experimental Psychiatry, 35*, 17–24.

Bienvenu, O. J., Samuels, J. F., Riddle, M. A., Hoehn-Saric, R., Liang, K. Y., Cullen, B. A., et al. (2000). The relationship of obsessive-compulsive disorder to possible spectrum disorders: results from a family study. *Biological Psychiatry, 48*, 287–293.

Blanchard, E. B., Andrasik, F., Neff, D. F., Arena, J. G., Ahles, T. A., Jurish, S. E., et al. (1982). Biofeedback and relaxation training with three kinds of headache: Treatment effects and their prediction. *Journal of Consulting and Clinical Psychology, 50*, 562–575.

Bordnick, P. S., Thyer, B. A., & Ritchie, B. W. (1994). Feather picking disorder and trichotillomania: an avian model of human psychopathology. *J Behav Ther Exp Psychiatry, 25*, 189–196.

Borkovec, T. D., & Costello, E. (1993). Efficacy of applied relaxation and cognitive-behavioral therapy in the treatment of generalized anxiety disorder. *Journal of Consulting and Clinical Psychology, 61*, 611–619.

Borkovec, T. D., Grayson, J. B., & Cooper, K. M. (1978). Treatment of general tension: Subjective and physiological effects of progressive relaxation. *Journal of Consulting and Clinical Psychology, 46*, 518–528.

Boudjouk, P. J., Woods, D. W., Miltenberger, R. G., & Long, E. S. (2000). Negative peer evaluation in adolescents: Effects of tic disorders and trichotillomania. *Child & Family Behavior Therapy, 22*, 17–28.

Brady, R. E., Diefenbach, G. J., Tolin, D. F., Hannan, S. E., & Crocetto, J. S. (2005, November). *What works in CBT for trichotillomania: Patients' self-report of efficacy*. Paper presented at the annual meeting of the Association for Behavioral and Cognitive Therapies, Washington, DC.

Brauer, A. P., Horlick, L., Nelson, E., Farquhar, J. W., & Agras, W. S. (1979). Relaxation therapy for essential hypertension. *Journal of Behavioral Medicine, 2*, 21–29.

Cardona, D., & Franklin, M. E. (2004). Help children and teens stop impulsive hair pulling. *Current Psychiatry, 3*, 73–76.

Carrion, V. G. (1995). Naltrexone for the treatment of trichotillomania: a case report. *J Clin Psychopharmacol, 15*, 444–445.

Carroll, L. J., & Yates, B. T. (1981). Further evidence for the role of stimulus control training in facilitation of weight reduction after behavioral therapy. *Behavior Therapy, 45*, 503.

Casati, J., Toner, B. B., & Yu, B. (2000). Psychosocial issues for women with trichotillomania. *Comprehensive Psychiatry, 41*, 344–351.

Chang, C. H., Lee, M. B., Chiang, Y. C., & Lu, Y. C. (1991). Trichotillomania: a clinical study of 36 patients. *J Formos Med Assoc, 90*, 176–180.

Chen, E., Touyz, S. W., Beumont, P. J., Fairburn, C. G., Griffiths, R., Butow, P., et al. (2003). Comparison of group and individual cognitive-behavioral therapy for patients with bulimia nervosa. *Int J Eat Disord, 33*, 241–254; discussion 255–246.

Christenson, G. A. (1995). Trichotillomania-from prevalence to comorbidity. *Psychiatric Times, 12*, 44–48.

Christenson, G. A., Chernoff-Clementz, M. A., & Clementz, B. A. (1992). Personality and clinical characteristics in patients with trichotillomania. *Journal of Clinical Psychiatry, 53*, 407–413.

Christenson, G. A., Crow, S. J., & Mackenzie, T. B. (1994, May). A placebo controlled double blind study of naltrexone for trichotillomania. *New Research Program and Abstracts of the 150th Annual Meeting of the American Psychiatric Association*, Philadelphia, PA, NR597.

Christenson, G. A., & MacKenzie, T. B. (1994). Trichotillomania. In M. Hersen & R. T. Ammerman (Eds.), *Handbook of prescriptive treatments for adults* (pp. 217–235). New York: Plenum.

Christenson, G. A., MacKenzie, T. B., & Mitchell, J. E. (1991a). Characteristics of 60 adult chronic hair pullers. *American Journal of Psychiatry, 148*, 365–370.

Christenson, G. A., MacKenzie, T. B., Mitchell, J. E., & Callies, A. L. (1991b). A placebo-controlled, double-blind crossover study of fluoxetine in trichotillomania. *American Journal of Psychiatry, 148*, 1566–1571.

Christenson, G. A., & Mansueto, C. S. (1999). Trichotillomania: Descriptive characteristics and phenomenology. In D. J. Stein, G. A. Christenson, & E. Hollander (Eds.), *Trichotillomania* (pp. 1–41). Washington, DC: American Psychiatric Press.

Christenson, G. A., & O'Sullivan, R. L. (1996). Trichotillomania: Rational treatment options. *CNS Drugs, 6*, 23–34.

Christenson, G. A., Pyle, R. L., & Mitchell, J. E. (1991). Estimated lifetime prevalence of trichotillomania in college students. *Journal of Clinical Psychiatry, 52*, 415–417.

Christenson, G. A., Raymond, N. C., Faris, P. L., McAllister, R. D., Crow, S. J., Howard, L. A., et al. (1994). Pain thresholds are not elevated in trichotillomania. *Biological Psychiatry, 36*, 347–349.

Christenson, G. A., Ristvedt, S. L., & MacKenzie, T. B. (1993). Identification of trichotillomania cue profiles. *Behaviour Research and Therapy, 31*, 315 320.

Clark, D. M., Salkovskis, P. M., Hackmann, A., Middleton, H., Anastasiades, P., & Gelder, M. (1994). A comparison of cognitive therapy, applied relaxation and imipramine in the treatment of panic disorder. *British Journal of Psychiatry, 164*, 759–769.

Cooper, J. (1970). The Leyton obsessional inventory. *Psychological Medicine, 1*, 48–64.

Cottraux, J., Gerard, D., Cinotti, L., Froment, J. C., Deiber, M. P., Le Bars, D., et al. (1996). A controlled positron emission tomography study of obsessive and neutral auditory stimulation in obsessive-compulsive disorder with checking rituals. *Psychiatry Research, 60*, 101–112.

Crocetto, J. S., Diefenbach, G. J., Tolin, D. F., & Worhunsky, P. (2003, November). *Trichotillomania and self-esteem.* Paper presented at the Annual Meeting of the Association for Advancement of Behavior Therapy, Boston, MA.

Deckersbach, T., Wilhelm, S., Keuthen, N. J., Baer, L., & Jenike, M. A. (2002). Cognitive-behavior therapy for self-injurious skin picking. A case series. *Behavior Modification, 26*, 361–377.

DeTore, N., D'Olio, C., Pasupuleti, R., Tolin, D., Diefenbach, G., Cahill, S., et al. (2006, November). Is there a relationship between pediatric trichotillomania and history of interpersonal violence? Poster to be presented at the Annual Meeting of the Association for Behavioral and Cognitive Therapies, Chicago, IL.

Diefenbach, G. J., Mouton-Odum, S., & Stanley, M. A. (2002). Affective correlates of trichotillomania. *Behaviour Research and Therapy, 40*, 1305–1315.

Diefenbach, G. J., Reitman, D., & Williamson, D. A. (2000). Trichotillomania: A challenge to research and practice. *Clinical Psychology Review, 20*, 289–309.

Diefenbach, G. J., Tolin, D. F., Crocetto, J. S., Maltby, N., & Hannan, S. E. (2005). Assessment of trichotillomania: A psychometric evaluation of hair pulling scales. *Journal of Psychopathology and Behavioral Assessment, 27*, 169–178.

Diefenbach, G. J., Tolin, D. F., Franklin, M. E., & Anderson, E. R. (2003, November). *The Trichotillomania Scale for Children (TSC): A new self-report measure to assess pediatric hair pulling.* Paper presented at the Annual Meeting of the Association for Advancement of Behavior Therapy, Boston, MA.

Diefenbach, G. J., Tolin, D. F., Hannan, S. E., Crocetto, J. S., & Worhunsky, P. (2004, May). *Trichotillomania: Impact on daily and quality of life.* Paper presented at the Annual Meeting of the *functioning* American Psychiatric Association, New York, NY.

Diefenbach, G. J., Tolin, D. F., Hannan, S., Maltby, N., & Crocetto, J. (2006). Group treatment for trichotillomania: Behavior therapy versus supportive therapy. *Behavior Therapy, 37*, 353–363.

Diefenbach, G. J., Tolin, D. F., Meunier, S. A., & Worhunsky, P. (2005, November). Emotion regulation and trichotillomania: A comparison of clinical and nonclinical hair pulling. In D. W. Woods (Chair), *Trichotillomania: Understanding relevant biobehavioral processes and derived treatments.* Symposium presented to the Annual Meeting of the Association for Behavioral and Cognitive Therapies, Washington, DC.

Dougherty, D. D., Rauch, S. L., & Jenike, M. A. (2002). Pharmacological treatments for obsessive compulsive disorder. In P. E. Nathan & J. M. Gorman (Eds.), *A guide to treatments that work* (2nd ed., pp. 387–410). New York: Oxford University Press.

du Toit, P. L., van Kradenburg, J., Niehaus, D. J. H., & Stein, D. J. (2001). Characteristics and phenomenology of hair-pulling: An exploration of subtypes. *Comprehensive Psychiatry, 42*, 247–256.

D'Zurilla, T. J., & Nezu, A. M. (1999). *Problem-solving therapy: A social competence approach to clinical intervention.* New York: Springer.

Eckstein, R. A., & Hart, B. L. (1996). Treatment of canine acral lick dermatitis by behavior modification using electronic stimulation. *J Am Anim Hosp Assoc, 32*, 225–230.

Epperson, N. C., Fasula, D., Wasylink, S., Price, L. H., & McDougle, C. J. (1999). Risperidone addition in serotonin reuptake inhibitor-resistant trichotillomania: Three cases. *Journal of Child and Adolescent Psychopharmacology, 9*, 43–49.

Fals-Stewart, W., Marks, A. P., & Schafer, J. (1993). A comparison of behavioral group therapy and individual behavior therapy in treating obsessive-compulsive disorder. *Journal of Nervous and Mental Disease, 181*, 189–193.

Faneslow, M. S. (1991). Analgesia as a response to aversive Pavlovian conditional stimuli: Cognitive and emotional mediators. In M. R. Denny (Ed.), *Fear, avoidance, and phobias: A fundamental analysis* (pp. 61–86). Hillsdale, NJ: Lawrence Erlbaum Associates.

First, M. B., Spitzer, R. L., Gibbon, M., & Williams, J. B. W. (1995). *Structured Clinical Interview for DSM-IV Axis I Disorders-Patient Edition (SCID I/P, version 2.0)*. New York: Biometrics Research Department.

Foa, E. B., & Kozak, M. J. (1997). Beyond the efficacy ceiling? Cognitive behavior therapy in search of theory. *Behavior Therapy, 28*, 601–611.

Fox, L. (1962). Effecting the use of efficient study habits. *Journal of Mathematics, 1*, 75–86.

Foxx, R. M., & Azrin, N. H. (1972). Restitution: a method of eliminating aggressive-disruptive behavior of retarded and brain damaged patients. *Behaviour Research and Therapy, 10*, 15–27.

Franklin, M. E., Abramowitz, J. S., Bux, D. A., Zoellner, L. A., & Feeny, N. C. (2002). Cognitive-behavioral therapy with and without medication in the treatment of obsessive-compulsive disorder. *Professional Psychology: Research & Practice, 33*, 162–168.

Franklin, M. E., & Foa, E. B. (2002). Cognitive-behavioral treatments for obsessive-compulsive disorder. In P. E. Nathan & J. M. Gorman (Eds.), *A guide to treatments that work* (2nd ed., pp. 367–386). New York: Oxford University Press.

Franklin, M. E., Foa, E. B., March, J. S. (2003). The Pediatric OCD Treatment Study (POTS): Rationale, design and methods. *Journal of Child and Adolescent Psychopharmacology, 13* (suppl. 1), 39–52.

Franklin, M. E., Keuthen, N. J., Spokas, M. E., Anderson, E., Tolin, D. F., Diefenbach, G. J., et al. (2002, September). *Pediatric trichotillomania: Descriptive psychopathology, comorbid symptomatology, and response to cognitive-behavioral treatment*. Presented to Maastricht, The Netherlands.

Franklin, M. E., Riggs, D. S., & Pai, A. (2005). Obsessive compulsive disorder. In M. M. Antony, D. Roth Ledley, & R. G. Heimberg (Eds.), *Improving outcomes and preventing relapse in cognitive-behavioral therapy* (pp. 128–173). New York: Guilford Press.

Franklin, M. E., Tolin, D. F., & Diefenbach, G. J. (2006). Trichotillomania. In E. Hollander & D. J. Stein (Eds.), *Clinical manual of impulse control disorders* (pp. 149–173). Washington, DC: American Psychiatric Press.

Frecska, E., & Arato, M. (2002). Opiate sensitivity test in patients with stereotypic movement disorder and trichotillomania. *Prog Neuropsychopharmacol Biol Psychiatry, 26*, 909–912.

Gluhoski, V. L. (1995). A cognitive approach for treating trichotillomania. *Journal of Psychotherapy Practice and Research, 4*, 277–285.

Golomb, R. G., & Vavrichek, S. M. (1999). *The Hair Pulling Habit & You*. Silver Spring, MD: Writers' Cooperative of Greater Washington.

Goodman, W. K., Price, L. H., Rasmussen, S. A., Mazure, C., Delgado, P., Heninger, G. R., et al. (1989). The Yale-Brown Obsessive Compulsive Scale. II. Validity. *Archives of General Psychiatry, 46*, 1012–1016.

Goodman, W. K., Price, L. H., Rasmussen, S. A., Mazure, C., Fleischmann, R. L., Hill, C. L., et al. (1989). The Yale-Brown Obsessive Compulsive Scale. I. Development, use, and reliability. *Archives of General Psychiatry, 46*, 1006–1011.

Graber, J., & Arndt, W. B. (1993). Trichotillomania. *Compr Psychiatry, 34*, 340–346.

Grachev, I. D. (1997). MRI-based morphometric topographic parcellation of human neo-cortex in trichotillomania. *Psychiatry and Clinical Neuroscience, 51*, 315–321.

Greist, J. H., Marks, I. M., Baer, L., Kobak, K. A., Wenzel, K. W., Hirsch, M. J., et al. (2002). Behavior therapy for obsessive-compulsive disorder guided by a computer or by a clinician compared with relaxation as a control. *Journal of Clinical Psychiatry, 63*, 138–145.

Guy, W. (1976). *Assessment manual for psychopharmacology.* Washington, DC: U.S. Government Printing Office.

Hall, S. M., & Hall, R. G. (1982). Clinical series in the behavioral treatment of obesity. *Health Psychology, 1*, 359–372.

Hanna, G. L. (1997). Trichotillomania and related disorders in children and adolescents. *Child Psychiatry and Human Development, 27*, 255–268.

Hannan, S. E., & Tolin, D. F. (2005). Mindfulness and acceptance based behavior therapy for obsessive-compulsive disorder. In S. M. Orsillo & L. Roemer (Eds.), *Acceptance and mindfulness-based approaches to anxiety: conceptualization and treatment* (pp. 271–299). New York: Springer.

Haugen, G. B., Dixon, H. H., & Dickel, H. A. (1963). *A therapy for anxiety tension reactions.* New York: Macmillan.

Hayes, S. C., Strosahl, K. D., & Wilson, K. G. (1999). *Acceptance and commitment therapy: An experiential approach to behavior change.* New York: Guilford Press.

Herrnstein, R. J. (1969). Method and theory in the study of avoidance. *Psychological Review, 76*, 49–69.

Hiss, H., Foa, E. B., & Kozak, M. J. (1994). Relapse prevention program for treatment of obsessive-compulsive disorder. *Journal of Consulting and Clinical Psychology, 62*, 801–808.

Holmbeck, G. N. , O'Mahar, K., Abad, M., Colder, C., & Updergrove, A. (2006). Cognitive-behavioral therapy with adolescents: Guides from developmental psychology. In P. C. Kendall (Ed.), *Child and adolescent therapy, third edition: Cognitive-behavioral procedures.* New York: Guilford Press.

Hollander, E. (1993). *Obsessive-compulsive-related disorders.* Washington, DC: American Psychiatric Press.

Iancu, I., Weizman, A., Kindler, S., Sasson, Y., & Zohar, J. (1996). Serotonergic drugs in trichotillomania: Treatment results in 12 patients. *Journal of Nervous and Mental Disease, 184*, 641–644.

Jacobson, E. (1929). *Progressive relaxation.* Chicago: University of Chicago Press.

Jenkins, J. R. (2001). Feather picking and self-mutilation in psittacine birds. *Veterinary Clin North Am Exot Anim Pract, 4*, 651–667.

Kabat-Zinn, J., Lipworth, L., & Burney, R. (1985). The clinical use of mindfulness meditation for the self-regulation of chronic pain. *J Behav Med, 8*, 163–190.

Keefer, L., & Blanchard, E. B. (2001). The effects of relaxation response meditation on the symptoms of irritable bowel syndrome: results of a controlled treatment study. *Behaviour Research and Therapy, 39*, 801–811.

Keijsers, G. P., van Minnen, A., Hoogduin, C. A., Klaassen, B. N., Hendriks, M. J., & Tanis-Jacobs, J. (2006). Behavioural treatment of trichotillomania: Two-year follow-up results. *Behaviour Research and Therapy, 44*, 359–370.

Kendall, P.C. (Ed.) (2006). *Child and adolescent therapy, third edition: Cognitive-behavioral procedures.* New York: Guilford Press.

Keuthen, N. J., Aronowitz, B., Badenoch, J., & Wilhelm, S. (1999). Behavioral treatment of trichotillomania. In In D. J. Stein, G. A. Christenson, & E. Hollander (Eds.), *trichotillomania (pp. 147–166).* Washington, DC: American Psychiatric Press.

Keuthen, N. J., Deckersbach, T., Wilhelm, S., Engelhard, I., Forker, A., O'Sullivan, R. L., et al. (2001). The Skin Picking Impact Scale (SPIS): scale development and psychometric analyses. *Psychosomatics, 42*, 397–403.

Keuthen, N. J., Fraim, C., Deckersbach, T., Dougherty, D. D., Baer, L., & Jenike, M. A. (2001). Longitudinal follow-up of naturalistic treatment outcome in patients with trichotillomania. *Journal of Clinical Psychiatry, 62*, 101–107.

Keuthen, N. J., Franklin, M. E., Bohne, A., Bromley, M., Levy, J., Jenike, M. A., et al. (2002, November). Functional impairment, interpersonal relatedness, and quality of life in trichotillomania. In N. J. Keuthen & M. E. Franklin (Chairs), *Trichotillomania: Psychopathology and treatment development.* Symposium presented to Reno, NV.

Keuthen, N. J., O'Sullivan, R. L., Ricciardi, J. N., Shera, D., Savage, C. R., Borgmann, A. S., et al. (1995). The Massachusetts General Hospital (MGH) Hairpulling Scale: 1. Development and factor analyses. *Psychotherapy and Psychosomatics, 64*, 141–145.

Keuthen, N. J., Savage, C. R., O'Sullivan, R. L., Brown, H. D., Shera, D. M., Cyr, P., et al. (1996). Neuropsychological functioning in trichotillomania. *Biological Psychiatry, 39*, 747–749.

Keuthen, N.J., Stein, D. J., Christenson, G.A. (2001). *Help for hair pullers: Understanding and coping with trichotillomania.* Oakland, CA, US : New Harbinger.

Keuthen, N. J., Wilhelm, S., Deckersbach, T., Engelhard, I. M., Forker, A. E., Baer, L., et al. (2001). The Skin Picking Scale: scale construction and psychometric analyses. *J Psychosom Res, 50*, 337–341.

King, R. A., Scahill, L., Vitulano, L. A., Schwab-Stone, M., Tercyak, K. P., & Riddle, M. A. (1995). Childhood trichotillomania: Clinical phenomenology, comorbidity, and family genetics. *Journal of the American Academy of Child and Adolescent Psychiatry, 34*, 1451–1459.

King, R. A., Zohar, A. H., Ratzoni, G., Binder, M., Kron, S., Dycian, A., et al. (1995). An epidemiological study of trichotillomania in Israeli adolescents. *Journal of the American Academy of Child and Adolescent Psychiatry, 34*, 1212–1215.

Koran, L. M., Ringold, A., & Hewlett, W. (1992). Fluoxetine for trichotillomania: An open clinical trial. *Psychopharmacology Bulletin, 28*, 145–149.

Koran, L. M., Thienemann, M. L., & Davenport, R. (1996). Quality of life for patients with obsessive-compulsive disorder. *American Journal of Psychiatry, 153*, 783–788.

Kovacs, M. (1985). The Children's Depression Inventory (CDI). *Psychopharmacology Bulletin, 21*, 995–998.

Kozak, M. J., & Foa, E. B. (1997). *Mastery of obsessive-compulsive disorder: A cognitive-behavioral approach.* San Antonio, TX: The Psychological Corporation.

Ladouceur, R. (1979). Habit reversal treatment: learning an incompatible response or increasing the subject's awareness? *Behaviour Research and Therapy, 17*, 313–316.

Ladouceur, R., Gosselin, P., & Dugas, M. J. (2000). Experimental manipulation of intolerance of uncertainty: a study of a theoretical model of worry. *Behaviour Research and Therapy, 38*, 933–941.

Lakein, A. (1973). *How to get control of your time and your life*. New York: Peter H. Wyden, Inc.

Lang, P. J. (1979). Presidential address, 1978. A bio-informational theory of emotional imagery. *Psychophysiology, 16*, 495–512.

Lenane, M. C., Swedo, S. E., Rapoport, J. L., Leonard, H., Sceery, W., & Guroff, J. J. (1992). Rates of Obsessive Compulsive Disorder in first degree relatives of patients with trichotillomania: a research note. *Journal of Child Psychology and Psychiatry, 33*, 925–933.

Leon, A. C., Olfson, M., Portera, L., Farber, L., & Sheehan, D. V. (1997). Assessing psychiatric impairment in primary care with the Sheehan Disability Scale. *International Journal of Psychiatry in Medicine, 27*, 93–105.

Leon, A. C., Shear, M. K., Portera, L., & Klerman, G. L. (1992). Assessing impairment in patients with panic disorder: The Sheehan disability scale. *Social Psychiatry and Psychiatric Epidemiology, 27*, 78–82.

Lerner, J., Franklin, M. E., Meadows, E. A., Hembree, E., & Foa, E. B. (1998). Effectiveness of a cognitive-behavioral treatment program for trichotillomania: An uncontrolled evaluation. *Behavior Therapy, 29*, 157–171.

Lilienfeld, S. O., Lynn, S. J., & Lohr, J. M. (2003). *Science and pseudoscience in clinical psychology*. New York: Guilford Press.

Linehan, M. M. (1993). *Skills manual for treating borderline personality disorder*. New York: Guilford Press.

Lovibond, S. H., & Lovibond, P. F. (1995). *Manual for the depression anxiety stress scales*. Sydney: The Psychology Foundation of Australia.

Maltby, N., Diefenbach, G. J., Tolin, D. F., Crocetto, J. S., & Worhunsky, P. (2004). *Quality of life assessment in the anxiety disorders: A psychometric evaluation*. Presented to the Annual Meeting of the Anxiety Disorders Association of America, Miami.

Maltby, N., & Tolin, D. F. (2005). A brief motivational intervention for treatment-refusing OCD patients. *Cognitive Behaviour Therapy, 34*, 176–184.

Manassis, K., Mendlowitz, S. L., Scapillato, D., Avery, D., Fiksenbaum, L., Freire, M., et al. (2002). Group and individual cognitive-behavioral therapy for childhood anxiety disorders: a randomized trial. *Journal of the American Academy of Child and Adolescent Psychiatry, 41*, 1423–1430.

Mansueto, C. S. (1990, November). *Typography and phenomenology of trichotillomania*. Paper presented at the annual convention of the Association for Advancement of Behavior Therapy, San Francisco, CA.

Mansueto, C. S., Stemberger, R. M. T., Thomas, A. M., & Golomb, R. G. (1997). Trichotillomania: A comprehensive behavioral model. *Clinical Psychology Review, 17*, 567–577.

March, J. S., Franklin, M., Nelson, A., & Foa, E. B. (2001). Cognitive-behavioral psychotherapy for pediatric obsessive-compulsive disorder. *Journal of Clinical Child Psychology, 30*, 8–18.

March, J. S., & Mulle, K. (1998). *OCD in children and adolescents: A cognitive-behavioral treatment manual*. New York, NY: Guilford Press.

March, J. S., Parker, J. D., Sullivan, K., Stallings, P., & Conners, C. K. (1997). The Multidimensional Anxiety Scale for Children (MASC): Factor structure, reliability, and validity. *Journal of the American Academy of Child and Adolescent Psychiatry, 36*, 554–565.

Marlatt, G. A. (1994). Mindfulness and metaphor in relapse prevention: An interview with G. Alan Marlatt. Interview by Deborah K. Shattuck. *J Am Diet Assoc, 94,* 846–848.

Marques, A. C., & Formigoni, M. L. (2001). Comparison of individual and group cognitive-behavioral therapy for alcohol and/or drug-dependent patients. *Addiction, 96,* 835–846.

Masters, J. C., Burish, T. G., Hollon, S. D., & Rimm, D. C. (1987). *Behavior therapy: Techniques and empirical findings* (3rd ed.). New York: Harcourt Brace Jovanovich.

Matson, J. L., Stephens, R. M., & Smith, C. (1978). Treatment of self-injurious behaviour with overcorrection. *J Ment Defic Res, 22,* 175–178.

Mayer, J. A., & Frederiksen, L. W. (1986). Encouraging long-term compliance with breast self-examination: the evaluation of prompting strategies. *J Behav Med, 9,* 179–189.

McElroy, S. L., Hudson, J. I., Pope, H., Jr., Keck, P. E., Jr., & Aizley, H. G. (1992). The DSM-III-R impulse control disorders not elsewhere classified: Clinical characteristics and relationship to other psychiatric disorders. *Am J Psychiatry, 149,* 318–327.

McKay, D. (1997). A maintenance program for obsessive-compulsive disorder using exposure with response prevention: 2-year follow-up. *Behaviour Research and Therapy, 35,* 367–369.

McKay, D., Todaro, J. F., Neziroglu, F., & Yaryura-Tobias, J. A. (1996). Evaluation of a naturalistic maintenance program in the treatment of obsessive-compulsive disorder: A preliminary investigation. *Journal of Anxiety Disorders, 10,* 211–217.

Meunier, S. A., Tolin, D. F., Diefenbach, G. J., & Brady, R. E. (2005, November). *Severity and course of hair pulling symptoms across the lifespan.* Paper presented at the Annual Meeting of the Association for Behavioral and Cognitive Therapies, Washington, DC.

Meunier, S. A., Tolin, D. F., & Franklin, M. E. (2005, November). *Affective and sensory correlates of hair pulling in a pediatric sample.* Paper presented at the Annual Meeting of the Association for Behavioral and Cognitive Therapies, Washington, DC.

Meyers, A. W., Thackwray, D. E., Johnson, D. B., & Schleser, R. (1983). A comparison of prompting strategies for improving appointment compliance of hypertensive individuals. *Behavior Therapy, 14,* 267–274.

Michelson, L., Mavissakalian, M., & Marchione, K. (1985). Cognitive and behavioral treatments of agoraphobia: Clinical, behavioral, and psychophysiological outcomes. *Journal of Consulting and Clinical Psychology, 53,* 913–925.

Miller, J. J., Fletcher, K., & Kabat-Zinn, J. (1995). Three-year follow-up and clinical implications of a mindfulness meditation-based stress reduction intervention in the treatment of anxiety disorders. *General Hospital Psychiatry, 17,* 192–200.

Miller, M. P., Murphy, P. J., & Miller, T. P. (1978). Comparison of electromyographic feedback and progressive relaxation training in treating circumscribed anxiety stress reactions. *Journal of Consulting and Clinical Psychology, 46,* 1291–1298.

Miller, W., & Rollnick, S. (2002). *Motivational interviewing: Preparing people for change* (2nd ed.). New York: Guilford.

Miltenberger, R. G., Fuqua, R. W., & McKinley, T. (1985). Habit reversal with muscle tics: Replication and component analysis. *Behavior Therapy, 16,* 39–50.

Mohr, D. C., Boudewyn, A. C., Goodkin, D. E., Bostrom, A., & Epstein, L. (2001). Comparative outcomes for individual cognitive-behavior therapy, supportive-expressive group psychotherapy, and sertraline for the treatment of depression in multiple sclerosis. *Journal of Consulting and Clinical Psychology, 69,* 942–949.

Mouton, S. G., & Stanley, M. A. (1996). Habit reversal training for trichotillomania: A group approach. *Cognitive and Behavioral Practice, 3*, 159–182.

Mouton-Odum, S., Keuthen, N. J., Wagener, P. D., Stanley, M. A., & DeBakey, M. E. (2006). StopPulling.com: An interactive, self-help program for trichotillomania. *Cognitive and Behavioral Practice, 13*, 215–226.

Murphy, M. T., Michelson, L. K., Marchione, K., Marchione, N., & Testa, S. (1998). The role of self-directed in vivo exposure in combination with cognitive therapy, relaxation training, or therapist-assisted exposure in the treatment of panic disorder with agoraphobia. *Journal of Anxiety Disorders, 12*, 117–138.

Nemeroff, C. B., & Schatzberg, A. F. (2002). Pharmacological treatments for unipolar depression. In P. E. Nathan & J. M. Gorman (Eds.), *A guide to treatments that work* (2nd ed., pp. 229–243). New York: Oxford University Press.

Ninan, P. T., Rothbaum, B. O., Marsteller, F. A., Knight, B. T., & Eccard, M. B. (2000). A placebo-controlled trial of cognitive-behavioral therapy and clomipramine in trichotillomania. *Journal of Clinical Psychiatry, 61*, 47–50.

O'Sullivan, R. L., Keuthen, N. J., Hayday, C. F., Ricciardi, J. N., Buttolph, M. L., Jenike, M. A., et al. (1995). The Massachusetts General Hospital (MGH) Hairpulling Scale: 2. Reliability and validity. *Psychotherapy and Psychosomatics, 64*, 146–148.

O'Sullivan, R. L., Rauch, S. L., Breiter, H. C., Grachev, I. D., Baer, L., Kennedy, D. N., et al. (1997). Reduced basal ganglia volumes in trichotillomania measured via morphometric magnetic resonance imaging. *Biological Psychiatry, 42*, 39–45.

Otto, M. W., Pollack, M. H., & Maki, K. M. (2000). Empirically supported treatments for panic disorder: costs, benefits, and stepped care. *Journal of Consulting and Clinical Psychology, 68*, 556–563.

Parks, G. A., Anderson, B. K., & Marlatt, G. A. (2001). Relapse prevention therapy. In N. Heather, T. J. Peters, & T. Stockwell (Eds.), *International handbook of alcohol dependence and problems* (pp. 575–592). New York: John Wiley & Sons.

Penzel, F. (2003). *The hair-pulling problem: A complete guide to trichotillomania.* New York: Oxford University Press.

Pollard, C. A., Ibe, I. O., Krojanker, D. N., Kitchen, A. D., Bronson, S. S., & Flynn, T. M. (1991). Clomipramine treatment of trichotillomania: A follow-up report on four cases. *Journal of Clinical Psychiatry, 52*, 128–130.

Prochaska, J. O., & DiClemente, C. C. (1982). Transtheoretical therapy: Toward a more integrated model of change. *Psychotherapy: Theory, Research, and Practice, 19*, 276–288.

Prochaska, J. O., DiClemente, C. C., & Norcross, J. C. (1992). In search of how people change. Applications to addictive behaviors. *American Psychologist, 47*, 1102–1114.

Rapoport, J. L., Ryland, D. H., & Kriete, M. (1992). Drug treatment of canine acral lick. An animal model of obsessive-compulsive disorder. *Arch Gen Psychiatry, 49*, 517–521.

Rapp, J. T., Miltenberger, R. G., Galensky, T. L., Ellingson, S. A., & Long, E. S. (1999). A functional analysis of hair pulling. *J Appl Behav Anal, 32*, 329–337.

Rapp, J. T., Miltenberger, R. G., & Long, E. S. (1998). Augmenting simplified habit reversal with an awareness enhancement device: Preliminary findings. *J Appl Behav Anal, 31*, 665–668.

Rapp, J. T., Miltenberger, R. G., Long, E. S., Elliott, A. J., & Lumley, V. A. (1998). Simplified habit reversal treatment for chronic hair pulling in three adolescents: A clinical replication with direct observation. *J Appl Behav Anal, 31*, 299–302.

Reeve, E. A. (1999). Hair pulling in children and adolescents. In E. Hollander (Ed.), *Trichotillomania* (pp. 201–224). Washington, DC: American Psychiatric Press.

Reeve, E. A., Bernstein, D. A., & Christenson, G. A. (1992). Clinical characteristics and psychiatric comorbidity in children with trichotillomania. *Journal of the American Academy of Child and Adolescent Psychiatry, 31*, 132–138.

Reinecke, M. A., Dattilio, F. M., & Freeman, A. (Eds.), (2003). *Cognitive therapy with children and adolescents: A casebook for clinical practice* (2nd edition, pp. 162–188). New York: Guilford Press.

Reinhardt, V., Reinhardt, A., & Houser, D. (1986). Hair pulling and eating in captive rhesus monkey troops. *Folia Primatol (Basel), 47*, 158–164.

Reiss, S., Peterson, R. A., Gursky, D. M., & McNally, R. J. (1986). Anxiety sensitivity, anxiety frequency and the prediction of fearfulness. *Behaviour Research and Therapy, 24*, 1–8.

Renjilian, D. A., Perri, M. G., Nezu, A. M., McKelvey, W. F., Shermer, R. L., & Anton, S. D. (2001). Individual versus group therapy for obesity: Effects of matching participants to their treatment preferences. *Journal of Consulting and Clinical Psychology, 69*, 717–721.

Rettew, D. C., Cheslow, D. L., Rapoport, J. L., Leonard, H. L., & Lenane, M. C. (1991). Neuropsychological test performance in trichotillomania: A further link with obsessive-compulsive disorder. *Journal of Anxiety Disorders, 5*, 225–235.

Romanczyk, R. G. (1974). Self-monitoring in the treatment of obesity: Parameters of reactivity. *Behavior Therapy, 5*, 531–540.

Romanczyk, R. G., Arnstein, L., Soorya, L. V., & Gillis, J. (2003). The myriad of controversial treatments for autism. In S. O. Lilienfeld, S. J. Lynn, & J. M. Lohr (Eds.), *Science and pseudoscience in clinical psychology* (pp. 363–395). New York: Guilford Press.

Rosenbaum, M. S., & Ayllon, T. (1981). The habit-reversal technique in treating trichotillomania. *Behavior Therapy, 12*, 473–481.

Rothbaum, B. O. (1992). The behavioral treatment of trichotillomania. *Behavioural Psychotherapy, 20*, 85–90.

Rothbaum, B. O., & Ninan, P. T. (1994). The assessment of trichotillomania. *Behaviour Research and Therapy, 32*, 651–662.

Rothbaum, B. O., & Ninan, P. T. (1999). Manual for the cognitive-behavioral treatment of trichotillomania. In D. J. Stein, G. A. Christenson, & E. Hollander (Eds.). *Trichotillomania.* Washington, D.C: American Psychiatric Press, Inc.

Rothbaum, B. O., Opdyke, D. C., & Keuthen, N. J. (1999). Assessment of trichotillomania. In E. Hollander (Ed.), *Trichotillomania* (pp. 285–298). Washington, DC: American Psychiatric Press.

Rothbaum, B. O., Shaw, L., Morris, R., & Ninan, P. T. (1993). Prevalence of trichotillomania in a college freshman population. *Journal of Clinical Psychiatry, 54*, 72–73.

Sanderson, K. V., & Hall-Smith, P. (1970). Tonsure trichotillomania. *Br J Dermatol, 82*, 343–350.

Schlosser, S., Black, D. W., Blum, N., & Goldstein, R. B. (1994). The demography, phenomenology, and family history of 22 persons with compulsive hair pulling. *Annals of Clinical Psychiatry, 6*, 147–152.

Scholing, A., & Emmelkamp, P. M. (1993). Exposure with and without cognitive therapy for generalized social phobia: Effects of individual and group treatment. *Behaviour Research and Therapy, 31*, 667–681.

Sheehan, D. V., Lecrubier, Y., Sheehan, K. H., Amorim, P., Janavs, J., Weiller, E., et al. (1998). The Mini-International Neuropsychiatric Interview (M.I.N.I.): The development and validation of a structured diagnostic psychiatric interview for DSM-IV and ICD-10. *Journal of Clinical Psychiatry, 59 Suppl 20*, 22–33;quiz 34 –57.

Simeon, D., Cohen, L. J., Stein, D. J., Schmeidler, J., Spadaccini, E., & Hollander, E. (1997). Comorbid self-injurious behaviors in 71 female hair-pullers: a survey study. *Journal of Nervous and Mental Disease, 185*, 117–119.

Simpson, H. B., Liebowitz, M. R., Foa, E. B., Kozak, M. J., Schmidt, A. B., Rowan, V., Petkova, E., Kjernisted, K., Huppert, J. D., Franklin, M. E., Davies, S. O., & Campeas, R. (2004). Post-treatment effects of exposure therapy and clomipramine in obsessive-compulsive disorder. *Depression & Anxiety, 19*, 225–233.

Smith, M. D., Haas, P. J., & Belcher, R. G. (1994). Facilitated communication: The effects of facilitator knowledge and level of assistance on output. *Journal of Autism and Developmental Disorders, 24*, 357–367.

Soriano, J. L., O'Sullivan, R. L., Baer, L., Phillips, K. A., McNally, R. J., & Jenike, M. A. (1996). Trichotillomania and self-esteem: A survey of 62 female hair pullers. *Journal of Clinical Psychiatry, 57*, 77–82.

Stangier, U., Heidenreich, T., Peitz, M., Lauterbach, W., & Clark, D. M. (2003). Cognitive therapy for social phobia: individual versus group treatment. *Behaviour Research and Therapy, 41*, 991–1007.

Stanley, M. A., & Cohen, L. J. (1999). Trichotillomania and obsessive-compulsive disorder. In D. J. Stein, G. A. Christenson, & E. Hollander (Eds.), *Trichotillomania.* Washington, DC: American Psychiatric Press.

Stanley, M. A., Borden, J. W., Mouton, S. G., & Breckenridge, J. K. (1995). Nonclinical hair-pulling: Affective correlates and comparison with clinical samples. *Behaviour Research and Therapy, 33*, 179–186.

Stanley, M. A., Breckenridge, J. K., Snyder, A. G., & Novy, D. M. (1999). Clinician-rated measures of hair pulling: A preliminary psychometric evaluation. *Journal of Psychopathology and Behavioral Assessment, 21*, 157–170.

Stanley, M. A., Hannay, H. J., & Breckenridge, J. K. (1997). The neuropsychology of trichotillomania. *Journal of Anxiety Disorders, 11*, 473–488.

Stanley, M. A., & Mouton, S. G. (1996). Trichotillomania treatment manual. In V. B. Van Hasselt & M. Hersen (Eds.), *Sourcebook of psychological treatment manuals for adult disorders* (pp. 657–687). New York: Plenum Press.

Stanley, M. A., Prather, R. C., Wagner, A. L., Davis, M. L., & Swann, A. C. (1993). Can the Yale-Brown Obsessive-Compulsive Scale be used to assess trichotillomania? A preliminary report. *Behaviour Research and Therapy, 31*, 171–177.

Stanley, M. A., Swann, A. C., Bowers, T. C., Davis, M. L., & Taylor, D. J. (1992). A comparison of clinical features in trichotillomania and obsessive-compulsive disorder. *Behaviour Research and Therapy, 30*, 39–44.

Stein, D. J., Christenson, G. A., & Hollander, E. (Eds.). (1999). *Trichotillomania.* Washington, DC: American Psychiatric Press.

Stein, D. J., Coetzer, R., Lee, M., Davids, B., & Bouwer, C. (1997). Magnetic resonance brain imaging in women with obsessive-compulsive disorder and trichotillomania. *Psychiatry Research, 74*, 177–182.

Stein, D. J., van Heerden, B., Hugo, C., van Kradenburg, J., Warwick, J., Zungu-Dirwayi, N., et al. (2002). Functional brain imaging and pharmacotherapy in trichotillomania. Single photon emission computed tomography before and after treatment with the selective serotonin reuptake inhibitor citalopram. *Prog Neuropsychopharmacol Biol Psychiatry, 26*, 885–890.

Stemberger, R. M. T., Thomas, A. M., Mansueto, C. S., & Carter, J. G. (2000). Personal toll of trichotillomania: Behavioral and interpersonal sequelae. *Journal of Anxiety Disorders, 14*, 97–104.

Stewart, R. S., & Nejtek, V. A. (2003). An open-label, flexible-dose study of olanzapine in the treatment of trichotillomania. *Journal of Clinical Psychiatry, 64*, 49–52.

Streichenwein, S. M., & Thornby, J. I. (1995). A long-term, double-blind, placebo-controlled crossover trial of the efficacy of fluoxetine for trichotillomania. *American Journal of Psychiatry, 152*, 1192–1196.

Stricker, J. M., Miltenberger, R. G., Garlinghouse, M. A., Deaver, C. M., & Anderson, C. A. (2001). Evaluation of an awareness enhancement device for the treatment of thumb sucking in children. *J Appl Behav Anal, 34*, 77–80.

Stuart, R. B. (1971). A three-dimensional program for the treatment of obesity. *Behaviour Research and Therapy, 9*, 177–186.

Sussman, N., & Stein, D. J. (2002). Pharmacotherapy for generalized anxiety disorder. In D. J. Stein & E. Hollander (Eds.), *Textbook of anxiety disorders* (pp. 135–139). Washington, DC: American Psychiatric Publishing.

Swedo, S. E., Lenane, M. C., & Leonard, H. L. (1993). Long-term treatment of trichotillomania (hair pulling) [Letter to the editor]. *The New England Journal of Medicine, 329*, 141–142.

Swedo, S. E., & Leonard, H. L. (1992). Trichotillomania. An obsessive compulsive spectrum disorder? *Psychiatric Clinics of North America, 15*, 777–790.

Swedo, S. E., Leonard, H. L., Rapoport, J. L., Lenane, M. C., Goldberger, E. L., & Cheslow, D. L. (1989). A double-blind comparison of clomipramine and desipramine in the treatment of trichotillomania (hair pulling). *The New England Journal of Medicine, 321*, 497–501.

Swedo, S. E., & Rapoport, J. L. (1991). Annotation: Trichotillomania. *Journal of Child Psychology and Psychiatry, 32*, 401–409.

Swedo, S. E., Rapoport, J. L., Leonard, H. L., Schapiro, M. B., Rapoport, S. I., & Grady, C. L. (1991). Regional cerebral glucose metabolism of women with trichotillomania. *Archives of General Psychiatry, 48*, 828–833.

Tarnowski, K. J., Rosen, L. A., McGrath, M. L., & Drabman, R. S. (1987). A modified habit reversal procedure in a recalcitrant case of trichotillomania. *Journal of Behavior Therapy and Experimental Psychiatry, 18*, 157–163.

Teng, E. J., Woods, D. W., Twohig, M. P., & Marcks, B. A. (2002). Body-focused repetitive behavior problems. Prevalence in a nonreferred population and differences in perceived somatic activity. *Behavior Modification, 26*, 340–360.

Tolin, D. F., Abramowitz, J. S., Brigidi, B. D., & Foa, E. B. (2003). Intolerance of uncertainty in obsessive-compulsive disorder. *Journal of Anxiety Disorders, 17*, 233–242.

Tolin, D. F., & Foa, E. B. (2001). Compulsions. In W. E. Craighead & C. B. Nemeroff (Eds.), *The Corsini encyclopedia of psychology and behavioral science* (3rd ed., pp. 338–339). New York: John Wiley & Sons.

Tolin, D. F., & Franklin, M. E. (2002). Prospects for the use of cognitive-behavioral therapy in childhood obsessive-compulsive disorder. *Expert Review of Neurotherapeutics, 2*, 89–98.

Tolin, D. F., Franklin, M. E., & Diefenbach, G. J. (2002, September). Cognitive-behavioral treatment of pediatric trichotillomania: An open trial. In A. Van Minnen (Chair), *Trichotillomania: Theory and treatment.* Symposium presented to the European Association of Behavioral and Cognitive Therapies, Maastricht, The Netherlands.

Tolin, D. F., Franklin, M. E., & Diefenbach, G. J. (2004, July). Cognitive-behavioral therapy for pediatric trichotillomania: An open trial. In J. Piacentini (Chair), *Treatment of childhood OCD and trichotillomania: New findings.* Symposium presented to the Annual Meeting of the American Psychological Association, Honolulu, HI.

Tolin, D. F., Franklin, M. E., Diefenbach, G. J., Anderson, E., & Meunier, S. A. (2006). Pediatric trichotillomania: Descriptive psychopathology and an open trial of cognitive-behavioral therapy. *Submitted for publication.*

Tolin, D. F., & Hannan, S. E. (2005). The role of the therapist in behavior therapy. In J. S. Abramowitz & A. C. Houts (Eds.), *Handbook of obsessive-compulsive spectrum disorders* (pp. 317–332). New York: Springer.

Tolin, D. F., & Hannan, S. E. (2005a). Mindfulness and acceptance based behavior therapy for obsessive-compulsive disorder. In S. M. Orsillo & L. Roemer (Eds.), *Acceptance and mindfulness-based approaches to anxiety: conceptualization and treatment* (pp. 271–299). New York: Springer.

Tolin, D. F., & Hannan, S. E. (2005b). The role of the therapist in behavior therapy. In J. S. Abramowitz & A. C. Houts (Eds.), *Handbook of obsessive-compulsive spectrum disorders* (pp. 317–332). New York: Springer.

Tolin, D. F., Maltby, N., Diefenbach, G. J., Hannan, S. E., & Worhunsky, P. (2004). Cognitive-behavioral therapy for medication nonresponders with obsessive-compulsive disorder: A wait-list-controlled open trial. *Journal of Clinical Psychiatry, 65*, 922–931.

Tolin, D. F., Maltby, N., Diefenbach, G. J., Hannan, S. E., & Worhunsky, P. (2004). Cognitive-behavioral therapy for medication nonresponders with obsessive-compulsive disorder: A wait-list controlled open trial. *Journal of Clinical Psychiatry, 65*, 922–931.

Turner, J. A. (1982). Comparison of group progressive-relaxation training and cognitive-behavioral group therapy for chronic low back pain. *Journal of Consulting and Clinical Psychology, 50*, 757–765.

Twohig, M. P., Hayes, S. C., & Masuda, A. (2006). A preliminary investigation of acceptance and commitment therapy as a treatment for chronic skin picking. *Behavior Research and Therapy, 44*, 1513–1522.

Twohig, M. P., & Woods, D. W. (2001a). Evaluating the duration of the competing response in habit reversal: a parametric analysis. *Journal of Applied Behavioral Analysis, 34*, 517–520.

Twohig, M. P., & Woods, D. W. (2001b). Habit reversal as a treatment for chronic skin picking in typically developing adult male siblings. *Journal of Applied Behavioral Analysis, 34*, 217–220.

van Minnen, A., Hoogduin, K. A., Keijsers, G. P., Hellenbrand, I., & Hendriks, G. (2003). Treatment of trichotillomania with behavioral therapy or fluoxetine. *Archives of General Psychiatry, 60*, 517–522.

van Nes, J. J. (1986). Electrophysiological evidence of sensory nerve dysfunction in 10 dogs with acral lick dermatitis. *Journal of the American Animal Hospital Association, 22*, 157–160.

Ware, J. E., & Sherbourne, C. D. (1992). The MOS 36-Item Short-Form Health Survey (SF-36): I. Conceptual framework and item selection. *Medical Care, 30*, 473–483.

Westen, D. (2000). The efficacy of dialectical behavior therapy for borderline personality disorder. *Clinical Psychology: Science & Practice, 7*, 92–94.

Wheeler, D. L., Jacobson, J. W., Paglieri, R. A., & Schwartz, A. A. (1992). *An experimental assessment of facilitated communication (TR #92-TA1)*. Schenectady, NY: OD Heck/ER DDSO.

White, S. D. (1990). Naltrexone for treatment of acral lick dermatitis in dogs. *J Am Vet Med Assoc, 196*, 1073–1076.

Winchel, R. M., Jones, J. S., Molcho, A., Parsons, B., Stanley, B., & Stanley, M. A. (1992). The Psychiatric Institute Trichotillomania Scale (PITS). *Psychopharmacology Bulletin, 28*, 463–476.

Winchel, R. M., Jones, J. S., Stanley, B., Molcho, A., & Stanley, M. A. (1992). Clinical characteristics of trichotillomania and its response to fluoxetine. *Journal of Clinical Psychiatry, 53*, 304–308.

Wong, L. (1994). *Essential study skills*. Boston, MA: Houghton Mifflin Company.

Woods, D. W., Flessner, C. A., Franklin, M.E. Keuthen, N. J., Stein, D., Goodwin, R. G., et al. (2006). Trichotillomania Impact Project (TIP): Exploring phenomenology, functional impact, and treatment utilization. *Journal of Clinical Psychiatry, 67*, 1877–1888.

Woods, D. W., & Miltenberger, R. G. (2001). *Tic disorders, trichotillomania, and other repetitive behavior disorders: Behavioral approaches to analysis and treatment*. Norwell, MA: Kluwer Academic Publishers.

Woods, D. W., Miltenberger, R. G., & Lumley, V. A. (1996). Sequential application of major habit-reversal components to treat motor tics in children. *J Appl Behav Anal, 29*, 483–493.

Woods, D. W., Wetterneck, C. T., & Flessner, C. A. (2006). A controlled evaluation of acceptance and commitment therapy plus habit reversal for trichotillomania. *Behaviour Research and Therapy, 44*, 639–656.

Wright, H. H., & Holmes, G. R. (2003). Trichotillomania (hair pulling) in toddlers. *Psychol Rep, 92*, 228–230.

Wynchank, D., & Berk, M. (1998). Fluoxetine treatment of acral lick dermatitis in dogs: a placebo-controlled randomized double blind trial. *Depress Anxiety, 8*, 21–23.

Yalom, I. D. (1995). *The theory and practice of group psychotherapy* (4th ed.). New York: BasicBooks.

INDEX

Printed in the United Kingdom
by Lightning Source UK Ltd.
123889UK00008B/82-84/A